どう行けば良いですか？
Nurse: We have a map on our website.
ホームページに地図が載っています。
Patient: OK. (I) (will) (check) it.
分かりました。確認します。

Dialog 2

Patient: Hello. I just called (a) (while) (ago)
こんにちは。少し前にお電話しました。
Nurse: Oh, yes. May I have your name?
あ、はい。お名前をお願いします。
Patient: My name is Brian Bachman.
ブライアン・バックマンと申します。
Nurse: Mr. Bachman, do you have health insurance?
バックマンさん、健康保険証はお持ちでしょうか？
Patient: (Here) (is) my Kokuminhoken card.
はい、国民保険証です。
Nurse: Please fill out this form.
こちらの書類を記入してください。
Patient: OK.
分かりました。
Nurse: Let me know if you have any trouble with it.
分からないことがあれば声をかけてください。

JN121051

Dialog 3

Nurse: Mr. Bachman?
バックマンさん。
Patient: Yes.
はい。
Nurse: This way please.
こちらへどうぞ。
Nurse: Please sit here.
こちらにお座りください。
Patient: (How) (long) will I have to (wait)?
どれくらい待たなければなりませんか？
Nurse: Your name will be called next.
次にお名前を呼びます。
Patient: OK. Thank you.
わかりました。ありがとうございます。
(moments later)
（しばらくして）
Nurse: Mr. Bachman. You may go in now.
バックマンさん、お入りください。

9. Listening Comprehension （巻末 Answer Sheet）

Dialog 1

Q1. What is the patient's problem?
患者はどこが悪いのか？
The patient has stomach pains.
患者は腹痛がある。

Q2.   How will he get to the clinic?
　　　 彼はクリニックへの道順をどのように見つけるか？
　　　 He will get to the clinic by checking the website.
　　　 彼はホームページを確認して医院へ行く。

Dialog 2

Q1.   Is the patient insured?
　　　 患者は健康保険に入っているか？
　　　 The patient is insured.
　　　 彼は保険に加入している。

Q2.   What did the nurse ask him to do?
　　　 看護師は彼に何をするよう言ったか？
　　　 The nurse asked him to fill out a form.
　　　 看護師は彼に用紙を記入するようお願いした。

Dialog 3

Q1.   When will the patient be called?
　　　 患者はいつ呼ばれるか？
　　　 He will be called next.
　　　 彼は次に呼ばれる。

QR コードで動画が見られる!

看護英語ワークブック

Answers
（解答編）

金芳堂

Lesson 1: Reception

ナースカナのワンポイントアドバイス

看護師は受付に出ることはそんなに多くはない。しかし、対応時は患者が身体的にも精神的にも不安を感じていることをお忘れなく。誠実かつ気配りのある対応で彼らの気持ちを和らげることが重要である。症状を見極め、手際よく患者を案内することが求められる。

1. Core Terms

1. nurse	2. appointment	3. problem	4. website	5. trouble
6. wait	7. ～と思われる	8. 腹痛	9. すぐに	10. 健康保険
11. 記入する	12. どれくらいの間～？		

4. Core Phrases

1. どうなさいましたか？
2. お名前をお願いします。
3. 健康保険証はお持ちでしょうか？
4. こちらの書類を記入してください。
5. 分からないことがあれば声をかけてください。
6. こちらへどうぞ。
7. こちらにお座りください。
8. お入りください。

6. Warm-up （巻末 Answer Sheet）／ 7. Workout with Julia

① (Go) (out) of the (west) exit of the station. (Turn) (left) and (go) (past) the hamburger shop. (Turn) (right) at the barber shop. (Walk) (straight) and you will find the clinic (on) (the) (right) (side).

② Go straight (along) the river. Turn east (at) the tall tree. (Go) (past) the shrine and turn right (at) the restaurant. (Go) (past) the police station and turn left (at) the hotel. The clinic is (on) (your) (left).

③ Kinpodo is located (north) (of) this clinic. Go out of the clinic and turn right. Next, turn right (at) (the) (front) of the hotel. Go straight and go past the police station. Turn right (at) (the) (corner) and (there) (will) (be) a school. Turn left and go straight. (You) (will) (find) Kinpodo on your left.

8. Dialogs

Dialog 1

Nurse: もしもし。かんやまクリニックです。

Patient: Hello. I don't have an (appointment).
もしもし。予約をしていませんが…

Nurse: What seems to be the problem?
どうなさいましたか？

Patient: I have (stomach) (pains).
腹痛があります。

Nurse: Is this your first visit to this clinic?
当院は初めてですか？

Patient: Yes, it is.
はい、そうです。

Nurse: Why don't you come over right now?
すぐに来院されてはどうでしょうか？

Patient: (How) (can) (I) (get) (there)?

Lesson 2: Patient Interview

ナースカナのワンポイントアドバイス

患者に関する情報は言語コミュニケーションを通じて得る。さらに、顔の表情、顔色、声質など非言語コミュニケーションを通じても患者の状態を知ることが出来ることも覚えておこう。患者の訴えに対して真摯に耳を傾ける態度を示すこと。そうすれば、彼らも話しやすくなる。また、プライバシーへの配慮もお忘れなく。

1. Core Terms

1. again	2. illness	3. hospital	4. before	5. currently
6. allergy	7. 深刻な	8. 肺炎	9. アキレス腱	10. 手術
11. 手術	12. 投薬	13. 症状	14. 吐き気	15. 嘔吐する

4. Core Phrases

1. 今までに重い病気に罹ったことはありますか？　2. 今までに手術を受けたことはありますか？

3. 今、お薬を服用していますか？　　　　　　　4. 何かアレルギーはありますか？

5. 特にどのあたりが痛みますか？　　　　　　　6. いつから痛み始めましたか？

7. 他に症状はありますか？

6. Warm-up

notepad　メモ帳	three color ballpoint pen　三色ボールペン
ruler　定規	scissors　ハサミ
surgical tape　テープ（ガーゼや点滴チューブを留める用）	tourniquet　駆血帯
watch　時計	hand sanitizer　手指消毒用スプレー
medical penlight　瞳孔ライト・ペンライト	personal seal　印鑑
alcohol swab　アルコール綿	calculator　電卓
bandage　絆創膏	

7. Workout with Julia

1. This is a notepad.	2. This is a three color ballpoint pen.	3. This is a ruler.
4. These are scissors.	5. This is surgical tape.	6. This is a tourniquet.
7. This is a watch.	8. This is hand sanitizer.	9. This is a medical penlight.
10. This is a personal seal.	11. This is an alcohol swab.	12. This is a calculator.
13. This is a bandage.		

8. Dialogs

Dialog 1

Nurse:　May I have your name again?
　　　　お名前をもう一度お願いします。

Patient: My name is Brian Bachman.
　　　　ブライアン・バックマンと申します。

Nurse:　Have you had any serious illnesses before?
　　　　今までに重い病気に罹ったことはありますか？

Patient: I was (in) (the) (hospital) with (pneumonia) last year.
　　　　昨年、肺炎で入院しました。

Nurse:　Have you ever had any operations before?
　　　　今までに手術を受けたことはありますか？

Patient: I (tore) my (tendon) and (had) (surgery) a few years ago.
　　　　数年前にアキレス腱を切って手術を受けました。

Nurse: Are you taking any medications currently?
          今、お薬を服用していますか？
Patient: No, I am not.
          いいえ。
Nurse: Do you have any allergies?
          何かアレルギーはありますか？
Patient: Yes, I am (allergic) (to) peanuts.
          はい。ピーナッツに対してアレルギーがあります。

Dialog 2
Nurse: What seems to be the problem?
          どうなさいましたか？
Patient: I am having (stomach) (pains).
          お腹の痛みがあります。
Nurse: Where does it particularly hurt?
          特にどのあたりが痛みますか？
Patient: The (lower) (right) (side) hurts.
          特に右下が痛いです。
Nurse: When did the pain start?
          いつから痛み始めましたか？
Patient: It started (this) (morning).
          今朝からです。
Nurse: Do you have any other symptoms?
          他に症状はありますか？
Patient: I have (nausea) and I (vomited) several times.
          吐き気があります。数回嘔吐しました。

9. Listening Comprehension（巻末 Answer Sheet）

Dialog 1
Q1.   What kind of illness did the patient have last year?
       患者が昨年患った病気は何ですか？
       The patient had pneumonia last year.
       患者は昨年肺炎に罹った。
Q2.   What kind of surgery did he have a few years ago?
       数年前に彼が受けた手術はどんなものですか？
       He had a surgery for a torn tendon.
       彼はアキレス腱断裂の手術を受けた。

Dialog 2
Q1.   Where is the pain?
       痛みはどこですか？
       The pain is in the lower right side.
       右の下腹部に痛みがある。
Q2.   What are the symptoms besides pain?
       痛み以外の症状は何ですか？
       The symptoms are nausea and vomiting.
       症状は吐き気と嘔吐である。

10. Vocabulary Test

1. again	2. illness	3. hospital	4. before	5. currently
6. allergy	7. serious	8. operation	9. medication	10. symptom

Lesson 3: Body Temperature and Pulse

ナースカナのワンポイントアドバイス

脈拍測定をすることは、患者の身体に直接触れることを意味する。患者を驚かさないよう、手が冷たくないか気を付けること。腕まくりをお願いする前にカーテンを引くなどプライバシーへの配慮を見せること。どのような処置を行うのか事前に説明すること。それにより不要な緊張を避けることができる。体温測定の際は、平熱を訊くことをお忘れなく。

1. Core Terms

1. date of birth	2. curtain	3. privacy	4. wrist	5. minute
6. normal	7. 体温	8. 体温計	9. 華氏	10. 摂氏
11. 速度	12. 脈拍	13. ～につき	14. ほんの少し	15. 緊張した

4. Core Phrases

1. 生年月日をお願いします。
2. 体温を測ります。
3. 体温計をもらえますか？
4. 平熱はどれぐらいですか？
5. 靴を脱いで横になってください。
6. カーテンを引きましょうか？
7. 手首をお願いします。
8. 緊張していますか？

6. Warm-up

1. Are you under a physician's care now? 今、お医者さんにかかっていますか？
2. Have you ever been hospitalized? 入院されたことはありますか？
3. Have you ever had a major operation? 大きな手術を受けたことはありますか？
4. Are you taking any medication now? 今、薬を服用していますか？
5. Are you on any special diet? 食事制限を受けていますか？
6. Do you use tobacco? タバコは吸いますか？
7. Do you drink alcohol? お酒は飲まれますか？

7. Workout with Julia

Are you under a physician's care now? 今、お医者さんにかかっていますか？
Case 1：Yes. はい。
Case 2：No. いいえ。

Have you ever been hospitalized? 入院されたことはありますか？
Case 1：Yes, I broke my leg and was hospitalized. はい、足を骨折して入院しました。
Case 2：Yes, my cold got worse and I got pneumonia. はい、風邪が悪化して肺炎になりました。

Have you ever had a major operation? 大きな手術を受けたことはありますか？
Case 1：Yes, for my broken leg. はい、骨折した足の。
Case 2：No. いいえ。

Are you taking any medication now? 今、薬を服用していますか？
Case 1：Yes, for my high blood pressure. はい、高血圧用で。
Case 2：Yes, for my cholesterol. はい、コレステロールの。

Are you on any special diet? 食事制限を受けていますか？
Case 1：Yes, I am on a low sodium diet. はい、塩分の制限をしています。
Case 2：Yes, I am on a low carb diet. はい、炭水化物ダイエット中です。

Do you use tobacco?　タバコは吸いますか？
Case 1：No, I don't.　いいえ、吸いません。
Case 2：Yes, one pack a day.　はい、1 日 1 パック。

Do you drink alcohol?　お酒は飲まれますか？
Case 1：Yes, I have some beers at night.　はい、夜にビールを少し。
Case 2：Yes, I have some cocktails before dinner.　はい、夕食前にカクテルを。

	Case 1	Case 2
1. Are you under a physician's care now?	はい。	いいえ。
2. Have you ever been hospitalized?	骨折で入院した。	肺炎で入院した。
3. Have you ever had a major operation?	その足の手術。	いいえ。
4. Are you taking any medication now?	高血圧の薬を。	コレステロールの薬を。
5. Are you on any special diet?	減塩ダイエット。	低炭水化物ダイエット。
6. Do you use tobacco?	いいえ。	1日1パック。
7. Do you drink alcohol?	晩にビール。	夕食前にカクテルを数杯。

8. Dialogs

Dialog 1
Nurse:　May I have your name?
　　　　お名前をお願いします。
Patient:　My name is Brian Bachman.
　　　　ブライアン・バックマンです。
Nurse:　May I have your date of birth?
　　　　生年月日をお願いします。
Patient:　My birthday is (February) (19th), (1980).
　　　　誕生日は 1980 年 2 月 19 日です。
Nurse:　OK.
　　　　はい。
Nurse:　I am going to take your temperature under your arm now.
　　　　わきの下で体温を測ります。
Nurse:　May I have the thermometer, please?
　　　　体温計をもらえますか？
Nurse:　Thank you. Your temperature is 36. 9.
　　　　ありがとうございます。体温は 36 度 9 分です。
Patient:　OK.
　　　　はい。
Nurse:　What is your normal temperature?
　　　　平熱はどれくらいですか？
Patient:　It is around (98) (degrees) Fahrenheit...which is about (36.6) (Celsius).
　　　　華氏で 98 度なので…摂氏 36.6 度くらいです。
Nurse:　I see. OK, we are finished, thank you.
　　　　分かりました。はい、終わりです。ありがとうございます。
Patient:　Thanks.
　　　　ありがとう。

Dialog 2
Nurse:　Please take off your shoes and lie down.
　　　　靴を脱いで横になってください。

Nurse: Shall I pull the curtain for privacy?
         プライバシーのためにカーテンをひきましょうか？
Patient: Yes, please.
         お願いします。
Nurse: Now I am going to take your pulse.
         これから脈を測ります。
Patient: OK.
         はい。
Nurse: May I have your wrist?
         手首をお願いします。
Patient: Here.
         はい。
Nurse: I am going to feel your pulse now...Just relax.
         では、脈を探します。楽にしてくださいね。
         (after one minute)
         （1分後）
Nurse: Your pulse rate is 100 beats per minute.
         あなたの脈拍は1分間に100回です。
Patient: Is that OK?
         それは、大丈夫ですか？
Nurse: It is a bit fast. Are you nervous?
         少し速いですね。緊張していますか？
Patient: (Maybe), (I) (am).
         そうかも。
Nurse: Between 60 and 100 is normal for an adult.
         大人の正常値は60から100の間です。
Patient: Oh, good. Thank you.
         よかった。ありがとう。

9. Listening Comprehension （巻末 Answer Sheet）

Dialog 1
Q1.   What is the patient's temperature?
      患者の体温は何度ですか？
      The patient's temperature is 36.9 degrees.
      患者の体温は36度9分である。
Q2.   What is the patient's normal temperature?
      患者の平熱は何度ですか？
      The patient's normal temperature is 36.6 degrees Celsius (98 degrees Fahrenheit).
      患者の平熱は摂氏36度6分（華氏98度）である。

Dialog 2
Q1.   What is the patient's pulse rate?
      患者の脈拍数はいくつですか？
      The patient's pulse rate is 100 beats per minute.
      患者の脈拍は1分間に100回である。
Q2.   What is the normal pulse rate for adults?
      成人の標準脈拍数はいくつですか？
      The normal pulse rate for adults is between 60 and 100.
      大人の脈拍正常値は60から100の間である。

10. Patient Interview ①

	箇所	症状
1	wrist／手首	sprained／捻挫 原因(階段から落ちた)
2	neck／首	stiff／凝っている 原因(自転車から落ちた)
3	stomach／胃	terrible stomachache／ひどい腹痛 原因(生魚を食べた)
4	right knee／右膝	原因(近所の犬に噛まれた)
5	ankle／足首	twisted／捻った 原因(サッカーをしていた)

Lesson 4: Blood Pressure

運動、入浴、食事は血圧に影響を与える。体が休まっているときに測定をする必要がある。血圧測定の前に、この点を確認すること。でなければ、再測定をすることになる…本レッスンのダイアログの動画と同じように。時には看護師の制服を見ただけで血圧が上昇する患者もいる。

1. Core Terms

1. take
2. table
3. second
4. squeeze
5. remove
6. uncross
7. 血圧
8. カフ（腕巻き）
9. 空気を入れる
10. 希望する
11. 普段
12. しばらくの間

4. Core Phrases

1. 血圧を測ります。
2. テーブルの上に腕を置いてください。
3. 腕にこのカフを巻きますね。
4. では今から空気を送り込みます。
5. 少しだけ腕を締め付けます。
6. カフを外します。

6. Warm-up

手
1. Show me your palm.　手のひらを見せてください。
2. Show me the back of your hand.　手の甲を見せてください。

腕
3. Straighten your arm.　腕をまっすぐ伸ばしてください。
4. Bend your arm.　肘を曲げてください。
5. Raise your arm.　腕を上げてください。
6. Put down your arm.　腕を下ろしてください。

足
7. Straighten your leg.　足をまっすぐにしてください。（寝ている状態）
8. Bend your knees.　膝を曲げてください。（寝ている状態）

全身
9. Please sit down.　座ってください。
10. Lie down with you head this way.　頭をこちらにして寝てください。（寝ている状態）
11. Please lie down facing the wall.　壁に向かって寝てください。（寝ている状態）
12. Please relax.　楽にしてください。

8. Dialogs

Dialog 1

Nurse:　I am going to take your blood pressure.
　　　　血圧を測ります。
Patient: OK.
　　　　はい。
Nurse:　Please put your arm on the table.
　　　　テーブルの上に腕を置いてください。
Patient: Sure.
　　　　わかりました。

Nurse:　I am going to place this cuff around your arm.
　　　　腕にこのカフを巻きますね。
　　　　Now, I am going to pump up the cuff.
　　　　では今から空気を送り込みます。
　　　　It will squeeze your arm just a little bit.
　　　　少しだけ腕を締め付けます。
　　　　But it will only be for a few seconds.
　　　　でも数秒だけです。
Patient:　(Go) (ahead).
　　　　どうぞ。
Nurse:　120 over 82.
　　　　上が 120、下が 82 ですね。
Patient:　(That) (sounds) (normal).
　　　　いつもそれくらいです。
Nurse:　I will remove this cuff.
　　　　カフを外します。

Dialog 2

Nurse:　Could you uncross your legs, please?
　　　　組んでいる足を戻してください。
Patient:　Oh, OK.
　　　　あ、はい。
Nurse:　Which arm do you prefer?
　　　　どちらの腕にしましょうか？
Patient:　Umm... (my) (right) (arm).
　　　　うーん。じゃ、右腕。
Nurse:　May I push up your sleeve?
　　　　袖をまくり上げていいですか？
Patient:　Sure.
　　　　ええ。
Nurse:　140 over 95.
　　　　上が 140 で下が 95 ですね。
Patient:　What?!
　　　　まさか?!
Nurse:　Is it usually this high?
　　　　普段もこの高さですか？
Patient:　It seems (higher) (than) (usual).
　　　　いつもより高い感じだな。
Nurse:　Did you do anything to raise your blood pressure?
　　　　血圧をあげるようなことをされましたか？
Patient:　I just (climbed) (the) (stairs) to this room.
　　　　ここへ来るときに階段を上りました。
Nurse:　OK, let's try it again 30 minutes later.
　　　　じゃ、もう一度 30 分後に測りましょう。
　　　　Please keep still for a while.
　　　　それまでしばらくじっとしていてください。
Patient:　Sure.
　　　　分かりました。

9. Listening Comprehension （巻末 Answer Sheet）

Dialog 1

Q1.   What did the nurse wrap around the patient's arm?
看護師は患者の腕に何を巻いたか？
The nurse wrapped a cuff around the patient's arm.
看護師は患者の腕にカフを巻いた。

Q2.   What was his blood pressure?
彼の血圧は？
His blood pressure was 120 over 82.
彼の血圧は最高血圧が 120、最低血圧が 82 であった。

Dialog 2

Q1.   What was the patient's blood pressure?
患者の血圧は？
The patient's blood pressure was 140 over 95.
患者の血圧は最高血圧が 140、最低血圧が 95 であった。

Q2.   Why was the blood pressure so high?
なぜ血圧がそんなに高いのか？
Because he just climbed the stairs.
彼が階段を上ってきたところだから。

10. Vocabulary Test

1. take	2. table	3. second	4. squeeze	5. remove
6. uncross	7. blood pressure	8. cuff	9. pump up	10. prefer

Lesson 5: Blood and Urine Sampling

血液採取は患者に痛みを伴う。だからこそ、一度で完了することが重要である。練習あるのみということをお忘れなく。体液の採取は患者の体調に関する情報を取得するのに重要である。したがって、これらのサンプルの取り扱いと管理には特別な注意を払う必要がある。尿の採取の場合は患者自身が行う。患者がそのやり方を正確に理解しているか確認すること。

1. Core Terms

1. pillow	2. straight	3. fist	4. thumb	5. visible
6. needle	7. 血管	8. 消毒する	9. 患部	10. わずかな
11. 痺れ	12. 吐き気	13. 尿	14. 容器	15. 残り

4. Core Phrases

1. この腕枕の上に腕を載せてください。
2. 腕を真っ直ぐ伸ばしてください。
3. 親指を中に入れて拳を作ってください。
4. 注射する所を消毒します。
5. 針を刺しますね。
6. 少しチクっとします。
7. では、針を抜きますね。
8. これを抑えて出血を止めてください。

7. Workout with Julia

	痛みの種類	痛みの場所
1	sharp　鋭い	（neck 首）
2	dull　鈍い	（back 腰）
3	stabbing　刺すような	（stomach お腹）
4	throbbing　ずきずきする	（head 頭）
5	burning　焼けるような	（chest 胸）
6	squeezing　締め付けるような	（chest 胸）
7	cramping　締め付けるような	（leg ふくらはぎ）
8	pounding　打たれるような	（head 頭）
9	shooting　打たれるような	（arm 腕）
10	splitting　割れるような	（head 頭）
11	tingling　ピリピリうずくような	（arm, skin 腕, 皮膚）
12	prickling　チクっとする	（arm, skin 腕, 皮膚）
13	nagging　しくしくする	（shoulder 肩）

8. Dialogs

Dialog 1

Nurse:　Mr. Bachman, I need to take some blood for a test.
　　　　バックマンさん。検査のために血液を採ります。

Patient: OK.
　　　　はい。

Nurse:　Put your arm on this pillow, please.
　　　　この腕枕の上に腕をのせてください。

Patient: Sure.
　　　　分かりました。

Nurse: Hold your arm out straight.
          腕を真っ直ぐ伸ばしてください。
Patient: (Like) (this)?
          このように？
Nurse: Yes. I will wrap this tourniquet around your arm.
          はい。この止血帯を腕に巻きます。
Nurse: Make a fist with your thumb inside to make your veins visible.
          親指を中に入れて拳を作ってください。血管を見やすくするために。
Patient: OK.
          はい。
Nurse: I will disinfect the site. It will feel a bit cold.
          注射する所を消毒します。ちょっと冷やっとします。
Nurse: I am going to put the needle in now.
          針を刺しますね。
Patient: (Will) (it) (hurt)?
          痛いですか？
Nurse: You will feel a slight pain.
          少しチクッとします。
Nurse: Do you feel any numbness or nausea?
          痺れや不快感はないですか？
Patient: No, I don't.
          いいえ。
Nurse: I am going to take the needle out now.
          では、針を抜きますね。
Nurse: OK. We are finished.
          はい、終わりです。
Patient: Pheew!
          ふー！
Nurse: Press on this to stop the bleeding.
          これを抑えて出血を止めてください。

Dialog 2

Nurse: We need to collect a urine sample, OK?
          検査のために尿を採取します。
Patient: Sure.
          はい。
Nurse: Here is the container.
          こちらが容器です。
Patient: (How) (should) (I) (fill) (it)?
          どのようにすればいいですか？
Nurse: First, pass a small amount of urine into the toilet.
          最初は少しおしっこをトイレに出してください。
Patient: I'll try.
          やってみます。
Nurse: Then start collecting your urine into the container.
          そのあとに容器におしっこを入れてください。
Patient: (How) (much) (do) (you) (need)?
          どれくらい必要ですか？
Nurse: Fill up to the line.
          線まで入れてください。

Patient: I see.
なるほど。
Nurse: After collecting the sample, pass the remaining urine into the toilet.
採取した後は、残りのおしっこをトイレに出してください。
Patient: OK.
分かりました。
Nurse: Also, do not touch the inside of the container.
また、容器の内側は触らないようにしてください。

9. Listening Comprehension

Dialog 1
Q1. How should the patient make his fist?
患者はどのようにして拳を作ればよいか？
The patient should make a fist with his thumb inside.
患者は親指を中に入れて握りこぶしをする。
Q2. What did the nurse do before inserting the needle?
針を入れる前に看護師は何をしたか？
The nurse disinfected the site.
看護師は注射部位の消毒を行った。

Dialog 2
Q1. What must the patient do first when collecting the urine?
尿を採取する際に患者はまず何をするべきか？
The patient must pass a small amount of urine into the toilet.
患者は便器に少量の尿を出す必要がある。
Q2. How much urine is necessary？　どのくらいの尿が必要か？
Up to the line (in the cup).　（コップの）線まで。

10. Patient Interview（2）

	症状
1	caught a cold／風邪を引いた 原因（上司から伝染された）
2	can't fall asleep／夜寝付けない 補足（朝まで羊を数えている）
3	appetite is gone／食欲がない
4	feel tired all the time／常に疲れている
5	trouble urinating／排尿しにくい

英会話コーナー 1

動画 4

Brian:　　　　What is your name?
　　　　　　あなたの名前は？

Julia:　　　　My name is Julia.
　　　　　　私の名前はジュリアです。
　　　　　　What is your name?
　　　　　　あなたの名前は？

あなた：　　　My name is (　　　　　).
　　　　　　私の名前は…です。
　　　　　　What is your name?
　　　　　　あなたの名前は何ですか？

Brian:　　　　My name is Brian Bachman.
　　　　　　私の名前はブライアン・バックマンです。

Brian & Julia:　Nice to meet you!
　　　　　　はじめまして！

動画 5

Julia:　　　Where do you live?
　　　　　どこに住んでますか？

Brian:　　　I live in Kyoto.
　　　　　京都に住んでいます。
　　　　　Where do you live?
　　　　　どこに住んでますか？

あなた：　I live in (　　　　　).
　　　　　…に住んでます。
　　　　　Where do you live?
　　　　　どちらに住んでいますか？

Julia:　　　I live in Osaka.
　　　　　大阪に住んでいます。
　　　　　How do you get to school?
　　　　　通学方法は？

あなた：　I get to school by (　　　　　).
　　　　　…で学校に行きます。
　　　　　How do you get to school?
　　　　　通学方法は？

Brian:　　　I get to school on roller skates.
　　　　　ローラースケートで学校に行きます。

Julia:　　　What?!
　　　　　何?!

動画 6

あなた：　What is your favorite food?
　　　　　好きな食べ物は？

Julia:　　　My favorite food is macaroni and cheese.
　　　　　私の好きな食べ物はマカロニ＆チーズです。
　　　　　What is your favorite food?
　　　　　あなたの好きな食べ物は？

あなた：　My favorite food is (　　　　　).
　　　　　私の好きな食べ物は…です。
　　　　　What is your favorite food?
　　　　　あなたの好きな食べ物は？

Brian:　　My favorite food is pizza.
　　　　　私の好きな食べ物はピザです。
　　　　　And my favorite topping is anchovies.
　　　　　そして、好きなトッピングはアンチョビです。
　　　　　What is your favorite topping?
　　　　　好きなトッピングは？

あなた：　My favorite topping is (　　　　　).
　　　　　私の好きなトッピングは…です。
　　　　　What is your favorite topping?
　　　　　好きなトッピングは？

Julia:　　I certainly love peperoni...but I can't stand anchovies!
　　　　　ペパロニがとても好きです…でも、アンチョビは許せないわ！

動画 7

Brian:　　What is your hobby?
　　　　　あなたの趣味は何ですか？

あなた：　My hobby is (　　　　　).
　　　　　私の趣味は…です。
　　　　　What is your hobby?
　　　　　あなたの趣味は何ですか？

Brian:　　My hobby is fishing.
　　　　　私の趣味は釣りです。

あなた：　What is your hobby, Julia?
　　　　　ジュリアさん、あなたの趣味は何ですか？

Julia:　　My hobby is having barbies.
　　　　　私の趣味はバービーです。

Brian:　　Barbie?
　　　　　バービー？
　　　　　Do you know what it is?
　　　　　それ何か分かりますか？

あなた：　No, I don't.
　　　　　分かりません。

Julia:　　It is what Americans call barbeque.
　　　　　アメリカ人が言うところのバーベキューですよ。

Brian:　　Hey! Why don't we have a barbeque this weekend?
　　　　　ねえ！週末みんなでバーベキューしようよ？

Julia:　　BARBIE!
　　　　　バービー！

Brian:　　Barbie...oh.
　　　　　バービー…あぁ。

Lesson 6: X-ray / Diagnosis

ナースカナのワンポイントアドバイス

診断結果を待っている間は患者にとってストレスのかかる時間である。深刻な病気があった場合、どうなるのだろうかと心配している。このストレスを最小限に抑えて、患者が落ち着くための時間を与えてから、医師と対面させること。したがって、患者の気持ちには注意を払い、絶えず気配りに努めること。

1. Core Terms

1. x-ray	2. stomach	3. metal	4. floor	5. judge
6. detail	7. 物体	8. 受付係	9. 虫垂炎	10. 炎症
11. 盲腸	12. 手術	13. 連絡する		

4. Core Phrases

1. お腹のレントゲンを撮りますね。
2. 金属類は身に着けないようにしてください。
3. 体内には金属類が入っていますか？
4. 必ずファイルを窓口に提出してくださいね。
5. 検査の結果あなたは虫垂炎になっています。
6. 手術をする準備をします。
7. お家に連絡のつく人はいますか？

6. Warm-up

1. 検査室　examination room
2. レントゲン室　x-ray room
3. 採血室　blood sampling room
4. 男性用トイレ　men's room
5. 女性用トイレ　women's room
6. 多目的トイレ　handicap toilet
7. 待合室　waiting room
8. 売店　store
9. 会計　cashier
10. 受付　reception

7. Workout with Julia

1. 検査室は廊下をまっすぐ進んで左に曲がってください。
2. レントゲン室へは、エレベーターで1階まで行ってください。
3. 採血室は向かって右側の3番目の部屋です。
4. 最も近い男性用トイレは角にあります。
5. 多目的トイレはエレベーターホールの近くにあります。
6. ご家族とはこの階の待合室でお会いになれます。
7. この階の待合室から電話をかけてください。
8. 売店は1階にあります。
9. 会計は1階の受付の横です。

8. Dialogs

Dialog 1 :

Nurse: Now we are going to take an x-ray of your stomach.
ではお腹のレントゲンを撮りますね。

Patient: OK.
はい。

Nurse: Make sure you do not have any metal objects on you.
金属類は身に着けないようにしてください。

Patient: Alright. I'll (take) (off) (my) (watch) and (necklace).
はい。時計とネックレスを外します。

Nurse: Do you have any metal objects inside your body?
体内には金属類は入っていますか？

Patient: What do you (mean) (by) (that) ?
どういうことですか？

Nurse:　For example, clips, stents, pacemakers....
例えばクリップやステントやペースメーカーなど。

Patient: Oh, I'm OK.
なるほど。大丈夫です。

Nurse:　Be sure to give this file to the receptionist.
必ずファイルを受付係に提出してくださいね。

Patient: So, how do I (get) (to) (the) (x-ray) (room) ?
で、レントゲン室はどこにありますか？

Nurse:　Please take the elevator to the first floor.
エレベーターで 1 階に降りてくださいね。

Patient: OK, thanks.
分かった。ありがとう。

Dialog 2 :

Doctor:　Mr. Bachman, judging from the tests, you have appendicitis.
バックマンさん、検査の結果あなたは虫垂炎になっています。

Patient: (What) (is) (that) ?
何ですか、それは？

Doctor:　It is inflammation of your appendix.
虫垂の炎症です。

Patient: Does it need to (be) (removed)?
取る必要があるのですか？

Doctor:　Yes, we will get ready for an operation this afternoon.
そうです。午後に手術をする準備をします。

Patient: Yipes!
ゲッ！

(moments later)
（しばらくして）

Nurse:　Is there anyone you can contact at home?
ご自宅に連絡のつく人はいますか？

Patient: Yes, (my) (wife) (is) (at) (home).
はい。妻が家にいます。

Nurse:　The doctor will explain the details to your wife.
先生が詳細について奥様に説明します。

Patient: OK. I will (call) (her).
分かりました。彼女に電話します。

9. Listening Comprehension （巻末 Answer Sheet）

Dialog 1

Q1.　What metal objects did the patient have on him?
どんな金属類を患者は身に着けていましたか？
The patient had a watch and necklace on.
患者は時計とネックレスを身に着けていた。

Q2.　How do you get to the x-ray room?
レントゲン室にはどのように行きますか？
You take the elevator to the first floor.
エレベーターで 1 階まで降りる。

Dialog 2

Q1.   What is the diagnosis?
　　　　診断結果は何ですか？
　　　　The diagnosis is appendicitis.
　　　　診断の結果は虫垂炎である。

Q2.   When will the operation take place?
　　　　いつ手術は行われますか？
　　　　The operation will take place in the afternoon.
　　　　手術は午後に行われる。

10. Vocabulary Test

1. x-ray   2. stomach   3. metal   4. judge   5. detail
6. receptionist   7. appendicitis   8. inflammation   9. appendix   10. operation

Lesson 7: Injection

ナースカナのワンポイントアドバイス

注射を安全に行うためには患者の協力が不可欠である。じっと座ってリラックスするように伝えること。多くの場合、注射は症状を和らげるために行われる。その時は、どれくらいで薬が効くかを説明すること。患者はこれにより安心する。注射の際、新人の方は遠慮なく先輩に同席してもらうのも良い。どんな時も冷静に。

1. Core Terms

1. still	2. prescribe	3. injection	4. relieve	5. allergic reaction
6. loosen	7. いくつかの	8. （痛みが）引く	9. すぐに	
10. アルコール消毒（消毒綿）		11. 右利き	12. ～の用意をする	
13. 痺れ	14. 微痛			

4. Core Phrases

1. 痛みを抑えるための注射をします。
2. お薬でアレルギーはありますか？
3. アレルギー反応を起こしたことはありますか？
4. あなたは右利きですか、左利きですか？
5. 左腕を見せてください。
6. 楽にして肩の力を抜いてください。
7. お薬を入れます。

7. Workout with Julia

1. 海老・全身に発疹 (shrimp / rashes all over my body)
2. 乳製品・息苦しい、時々意識がなくなる (dairy products / trouble breathing, sometimes I pass out)
3. ハウスダスト・肌が赤くなる (house dust, dust mites / skin gets red)
4. 抗生剤・発疹、痒み (antibiotics / rashes, itchiness)
5. アスピリン・ひどい咳 (aspirin / coughing badly)
6. ピーナッツ・息苦しい (peanut / trouble breathing)
7. 花粉症・くしゃみ、咳、目の痒み (hay fever / sneezing, coughing, and itchy eyes)
8. リドカイン・咳、息苦しい (lidocaine / coughing, trouble breathing)
9. ペット・咳、ひどい目の痒み (pets / coughing, my eyes itch a lot)
10. 卵・吐き気、嘔吐 (egg / nausea, vomit)

8. Dialogs

Dialog 1

Nurse: Mr. Bachman? Do you still have stomach pains?
　　　　バックマンさん、まだ腹痛はありますか？

Patient: Yes, (very) (much).
　　　　はい。まだとても痛いです。

Nurse: The doctor will prescribe an injection for the pain.
　　　　先生が痛みを抑える注射を処方しますよ。

Patient: But, but...I (don't) (like) (shots).
　　　　え、え、でも…注射は苦手です。

Nurse: Don't worry, it will be over in a couple of seconds.
　　　　ご心配なく。数秒で終わりますよ。

Patient: OK. How soon will it (relieve) (the) (pain)?
　　　　分かりました。痛みはどれくらいで引きますか？

Nurse: The pain should start to subside immediately.
　　　　痛みはすぐに引き始めます。

Dialog 2

Nurse: I will give you an injection to relieve the pain.
          痛みを抑えるための注射をします。
Brian: Uh, OK.
          あ、はい。
Nurse: Are you allergic to any medication?
          お薬でアレルギーはありますか？
Brian: No, I am not.
          いいえ。ありません。
Nurse: Have you experienced any allergic reactions to alcohol wipes?
          アルコール消毒（消毒綿）でアレルギー反応を起こしたことはありますか？
Patient: No, I haven't.
          いいえ、ありません。
Nurse: Are you right handed or left handed?
          あなたは右利きですか、左利きですか？
Patient: (I) (am) (right) (handed).
          私は右利きです。
Nurse: May I see your left arm?
          左腕を見せてください。
Nurse: It looks OK. I will get ready for the injection.
          いいですね。では注射の用意をします。
Nurse: Please relax and loosen your shoulders.
          では、楽にして肩の力を抜いてください。
Patient: OK.
          はい。
Nurse: You will feel a slight pain.
          すこしチクッとします。
Nurse: Do you feel any numbness or tingling?
          しびれや電気が走る感じがしますか？
Patient: No.
          いいえ。
Nurse: OK. I will inject the medication.
          はい。お薬を入れます。
Nurse: We are finished.
          はい。終わりました。
Nurse: I will remove the needle.
          では、針を抜きますね。
Nurse: Press on this to stop the bleeding.
          これを抑えて血を止めます。
Patient: Thanks.
          ありがとう。

9. Listening Comprehension （巻末 Answer Sheet）

Dialog 1

Q1.   What will the doctor prescribe for the pain?
       痛みを止めるために医師は何を処方しますか？
       The doctor will prescribe an injection for the pain.
       医師は痛み止めの注射を処方する。
Q2.   How soon will the pain subside?
       どれくらいで痛みは引きますか？

The pain will start to subside immediately.
痛みはすぐに引き始める。

Dialog 2

Q1.   Does the patient have any allergies?
       患者は何らかのアレルギーを持っていますか？
       The patient does not have any allergies.
       患者はアレルギーがない。

Q2.   Which arm did the nurse inject the medication?
       どちらの腕に看護師は薬を注射しましたか？
       The nurse injected the medication in the left arm.
       看護師は左腕に注射をした。

10. Patient Interview（3）

	箇所	症状
1		dizzy／めまい 補足（座らないといけない）
2	throat／喉	lump／できもの 補足（物を飲み込みにくい）
3		原因（蛇に噛まれた）
4	pelvis／骨盤	pain／痛み
5	sinus／鼻腔	congested／鼻づまり 補足（息がしにくい）

Lesson 8: Concerning the Operation

ナースカナのワンポイントアドバイス

手術の前、患者は痛みを伴うか、どれくらい時間がかかるか、いつ仕事に復帰できるかを心配している。これらの不透明な状況は、大きな不安の原因となる。この負担を軽減するためには、患者からのどのような質問にも対応することが私たちの責務である。

1. Core Terms

1. operation	2. explain	3. nervous	4. sign	5. question
6. take a shower	7. 麻酔	8. ほっとする	9. 処置	10. 同意書
11. ～に関する	12. 円滑に	13. お粥	14. 拭う	

4. Core Phrases

1. ご気分はいかがですか？
2. 麻酔がかかっていますよ。
3. 痛みは感じません。
4. 同意書にサインをする必要があります。
5. 日本語は読めますか？
6. 説明に関して何か質問はありますか？

7. Workout with Julia

Case 1. 痛み／昨夜／断続的
Case 2. 痒み／昨晩の夕食後／その他（数時間続いたが、今は大丈夫）
Case 3. めまい／先週／断続的（朝と立ち上がった時）
Case 4. 吐き気／今朝／持続的（朝食が喉を通らない）
Case 5. 咳／先週／断続的（朝起きた時が一番ひどい）
Case 6. 倦怠感／数か月間／持続的

8. Dialogs

Dialog 1

Nurse: Mr. Bachman. So, how do you feel?
バックマンさん、ご気分はいかがですか？
Patient: I'm kind of (nervous).
緊張しています。
Nurse: Don't worry.
心配しないで。
Patient: I'm trying not to. Will it (hurt)?
しないようにしていますが。痛みますか？
Nurse: You'll be under anesthesia, so you won't feel anything.
麻酔にかかっていますので、何も感じませんよ。
Patient: OK. I'm a bit (relieved) to hear that.
分かりました。それを聞いて少しホッとしました。
Nurse: Before starting the procedures, you need to sign a consent form.
手術の前に、同意書に署名をする必要があります。
Patient: No problem.
いいですよ。
Nurse: So, here is the form. Can you read Japanese?
では、こちらが同意書です。日本語は読めますか？
Patient: Uh, no....
えっと、いえ…。
Nurse: OK. Here's what it says....
分かりました。こう書かれています…。

Dialog 2

Nurse: Do you have any questions concerning the explanations?
         説明に関して何か質問はありますか？

Patient: Yes, I do. When can I (start) (eating) after the operation?
         あります。手術後はいつ食事を始めることができますか？

Nurse: If everything goes smoothly, you can eat lunch tomorrow.
         予定通りいきますと、明日のお昼ごはんから食べれます。

Patient: (What) (kind) (of) food can I eat?
         どのような食事ができますか？

Nurse: For tomorrow, you can only eat rice porridge.
         明日のところは、お粥しか食べれません。

Patient: When can I (take) (a) (shower)?
         シャワーはいつ浴びれますか？

Nurse: Not tomorrow.
         明日は無理です。

Patient: Oh....
         あらぁ…。

Nurse: I will wipe your body. You can start taking showers from the day after tomorrow.
         私が体を拭きます。明後日からシャワーを浴びることができます。

9. Listening Comprehension （巻末 Answer Sheet）

Dialog 1

Q1.   What is the patient worried about?
      患者は何を心配していますか？
      The patient is worried if it will hurt.
      患者は痛みを伴うか心配している。

Q2.   What does the patient need to sign before the operation?
      手術の前に患者は何に署名しなければいけませんか？
      The patient needs to sign a consent form.
      患者は同意書に署名する必要がある。

Dialog 2

Q1.   When can the patient start eating?
      いつから患者は食べることが出来ますか？
      The patient can start eating from lunch tomorrow.
      患者は明日の昼食から食事を始めることができる。

Q2.   What will the patient eat on the next day after the operation?
      手術の翌日に患者は何を食べますか？
      The patient will eat rice porridge.
      患者はお粥を食べる。

10. Vocabulary Test

1. operation	2. explain	3. nervous	4. sign	5. question
6. anesthesia	7. consent form	8. concerning	9. smoothly	10. wipe

Lesson 9: After the Operation

食事に関する指導も看護師の業務の一部である。検査や手術の前後に食事の制限があることを説明しなくてはいけない。例えば、塩分の制限、場合によっては絶食を伴うこともあります。さらに、リハビリがどれくらい続くかを知らせることにより、患者を勇気づけてより良い結果をもたらすことが出来る。

1. Core Terms

1. vein
2. tight
3. relax
4. juice
5. soup
6. fruit
7. add
8. 点滴
9. 挿入する
10. 液体
11. 少し
12. 駆血帯
13. 消化
14. 焼く

4. Core Phrases

1. 今から点滴をします。
2. 小さなプラスチックの管を血管に挿入します。
3. 水分を補うために必要です。
4. 駆血帯を巻きます。
5. きつ過ぎたら言ってください。

7. Workout with Julia

Part 1

1. This is a stethoscope. 聴診器
2. These are exam gloves. グローブ
3. This is a blood pressure monitor. 血圧計
4. This is an electronic thermometer. 電子体温計
5. This is a cotton swab. 綿棒（商品名 Q-tip とも言う）
6. This is a dressing. 包帯
7. This is saline. 生理食塩水
8. These are tweezers. 鑷子（せっし）
9. This is a kidney tray. 膿盆
10. This is a syringe. 注射器
11. This is a sharps disposal. 針捨て容器
12. This is a tongue depressor. 舌圧子

Part 2

1. stethoscope
2. blood pressure monitor
3. tweezers
4. syringe

8. Dialogs

Dialog 1

Nurse: I need to give you an intravenous infusion.
今から点滴をします。
Patient: How are you going (to) (do) (it)?
どのようにするのですか？
Nurse: A small plastic tube is inserted into your vein.
小さなプラスチックの管を挿入します。
Patient: I see.
なるほど。
Nurse: It is necessary to give you fluids.
水分を与えるために必要です。
Patient: Will it be (painful)?
痛みますか？
Nurse: There is only a slight pain at the beginning.
最初に少しチクッとするだけです。
Nurse: I am going to put a tourniquet on.
駆血帯を巻きます。
Nurse: If it is too tight, let me know.

きつ過ぎたら言ってください。
Patient: I am OK.
　　　　大丈夫です。
　　　　(all set)
　　　　（セッティング完了）
Nurse:　Is everything OK?
　　　　どうですか。
Patient: I feel (fine).
　　　　大丈夫です。

Dialog 2

Patient: So, what (will) (I) (be) eating here?
　　　　ここではどのような食事が出るのですか？
Nurse:　You will be eating foods that help digestion.
　　　　消化に良い物を食べることになります。
Patient: What kind of food (would) (that) (be)?
　　　　どのような食べ物ですか？
Nurse:　You will start off with rice porridge, soup, and juice.
　　　　最初はお粥やスープやジュースです。
Patient: I see.
　　　　なるほど。
Nurse:　From day 3, rice, broiled fish, potato salad and canned fruit will be added to the menu.
　　　　3日目からごはん、焼き魚、ポテトサラダ、缶詰のフルーツなどがでます。
Patient: Oh boy, I can't wait!
　　　　いいね。待ちきれない！

9. Listening Comprehension （巻末 Answer Sheet）

Dialog 1

Q1.　　How did the nurse explain an intravenous infusion?
　　　　看護師は点滴についてどのように説明しましたか？
　　　　A small plastic tube will be inserted into the vein.
　　　　小さいプラスチックの管が血管に挿入される。
Q2.　　Why is the intravenous infusion necessary?
　　　　なぜ点滴が必要なのか？
　　　　It is necessary to give the patient fluids.
　　　　患者に水分補給をするために必要である。

Dialog 2

Q1.　　What kind of food will the patient eat?
　　　　患者はどのような食事をしますか？
　　　　The patient will eat foods that help digestion.
　　　　患者は消化しやすい食べ物を食べる。
Q2.　　What kind of food will the patient eat from day 3?
　　　　患者は3日目からどのような食事をしますか？
　　　　The patient will eat rice, broiled fish, potato salad, and canned fruit.
　　　　患者はご飯、焼き魚、ポテトサラダ、缶詰のフルーツを食べる。

10. Patient Interview ⑷

	箇所	症状
1	left ear／左耳	trouble hearing／聞きづらい
2	shoulder／肩	pain ／痛み 補足（腕を挙げると）
3	all over the body／全身	rashes ／発疹 itch ／痒い
4		blood mixed in his stool／血便
5		diarrhea／下痢 補足（今朝から）

Lesson 10: Dry Bath

清拭は患者さんの体を清潔にすることだけではない。患者さんの体に関する重要な情報を得る機会だ。体に触れることで、熱はないか、発疹や腫れはないか、皮膚は乾燥していないか、床ずれはできていないかを確認することが出来る。これらの情報を医師に報告し、情報を必要な看護に活用することができる。ただし、羞恥心を伴うケアになるので、十分に注意すること。

1. Core Terms

1. towel
2. schedule
3. rehabilitation
4. shirt
5. stitch
6. itch
7. 正しい
8. 脱ぐ
9. 湿疹
10. お腹
11. 外科用テープ

4. Core Phrases

1. 前に説明したとおり、清拭はできますよ。
2. 熱いタオルで体を拭きます。
3. リハビリの後にしましょう。
4. 熱すぎませんか？
5. シャツを脱いでもらえますか？
6. 先生に診てもらいます。

7. Workout with Julia

Case 1. 左ひざの関節／鋭い痛み (joint of my left knee / sharp pain)
Case 2. のど／焼けるような痛み (throat / burning pain)
Case 3. 副鼻腔／鈍い痛み (sinus / dull pain)
Case 4. 腰／継続的な鈍い痛み (back / constant dull pain)
Case 5. 頭／ずきずきする痛み (headache / throbbing pain)
Case 6. 下腹部／ひきつけるような痛み (abdomen / cramping pain)
Case 7. 胸／締め付けられるような痛み (chest / squeezing pain)
Case 8. 右肩／しつこい痛み (right shoulder / nagging pain)

8. Dialogs

Dialog 1

Patient: So I can't (take) (a) (shower) today, right?
で、シャワーは浴びれないんですよね？

Nurse: That's correct. You just had an operation.
そうですね。手術したばかりなので。
Like I explained before, I can give you a dry bath.
以前にも説明したように、清拭をします。

Patient: What was that?
それって何でした？

Nurse: I will wipe your body with a hot towel.
熱いタオルで体を拭きます。

Patient: Oh yes, right! Good idea...but I am (scheduled) (for) (rehab).
そうだった！いい考えだけど…でもリハビリの予定が入っています。

Nurse: No problem. Let's do it after your rehabilitation.
大丈夫です。リハビリの後にしましょう。

Dialog 2

Nurse: I will wipe your body.
体をお拭きします。

Patient: Great.

お願いします。

Nurse:　May I have your arm? Is it too hot?
腕を出していただけますか？熱すぎませんか？

Patient:　No, it's (just) (right).
いいえ、ちょうど良いです。

Nurse:　Can you take your gown off?
ガウンを脱いでいただけますか？

Patient:　I'll try...Oooh! (My) (stitches) (hurt).
やってみるけど…あぁ！縫ったところが痛い。

Nurse:　OK. I'll help you.
分かりました。手伝います。
(moments later)
しばらくして

Nurse:　Hmmmm. You have rashes on your tummy. Does it itch?
んー。お腹に湿疹がありますね。痒いですか？

Patient:　No, it doesn't.
いいえ。

Nurse:　It probably got red from the surgical tape. I'll have the doctor check it.
おそらくテープで赤くなったのでしょう。先生に診てもらいます。

Patient:　Thanks.
ありがとう。
(moments later)
しばらくして

Patient:　Wow. I feel (refreshed).
わぁ。すっきりした。

9. Listening Comprehension （巻末 Answer Sheet）

Dialog 1
Q1.　How will the nurse give a dry bath?
看護師はどのように清拭を行いますか？
The nurse will wipe the patient's body with a hot towel.
看護師は熱いタオルで患者の体を拭く。

Q2.　When will she give the patient the dry bath?
看護師はいつ清拭を行いますか？
She will give the dry bath after the rehabilitation.
彼女はリハビリ後に清拭を行う。

Dialog 2
Q1.　What did the patient have on his stomach?
患者のお腹には何がありましたか？
The patient had rashes on his stomach.
患者はお腹に湿疹ができていた。

Q2.　What probably caused it?
何がおそらくそれを引き起こしましたか？
It was probably caused by the surgical tape.
おそらく外科用テープが原因であった。

10. Vocabulary Test

1. towel
2. schedule
3. rehabilitation
4. shirt
5. stitch
6. itch
7. correct
8. rash
9. tummy
10. surgical tape

英会話コーナー 2

動画 4

Julia:　　　　Are you healthy?
　　　　　　　あなたは健康ですか？

あなた：　　　Yes, I am healthy. / No, I am not healthy.
　　　　　　　私は健康です。／私は不健康です。
　　　　　　　Are you healthy?
　　　　　　　あなたは健康ですか？

Julia:　　　　Yes, I am. How about you Brian.
　　　　　　　はい、健康です。ブライアン、あなたはどう？

Brian:　　　　I am not healthy.
　　　　　　　私は不健康です。

あなた：　　　Why are you not healthy?
　　　　　　　何で不健康なのですか？

Brian:　　　　I haven't been sleeping at all.
　　　　　　　しっかり眠れていません。

あなた：　　　How many hours do you sleep?
　　　　　　　あなたの睡眠時間は？

Brian:　　　　I sleep about 5 hours.
　　　　　　　およそ 5 時間です。

Julia:　　　　That is short.
　　　　　　　短いですね。
　　　　　　　What about you?
　　　　　　　あなたはどうなの？

あなた：　　　I sleep about (　　　　　　) hours.
　　　　　　　私は約…時間寝ます。

Brian and Julia: I see.
　　　　　　　そうなんだ。

動画 5

あなた：How tall are you, Julia?
　　　　ジュリアさん、あなたの身長は？

Julia:　I am 165 centimeters tall.
　　　　私は 165cm です。
　　　　So, how tall are you?
　　　　で、あなたの身長は？

あなた：I am @@@ centimeters tall.
　　　　私の身長は…センチです。
　　　　How tall are you, Brian?
　　　　ブライアンさん、あなたの身長は？

Brian:　I am 190 centimeters and still growing.
　　　　私は 190 センチで、まだ伸びてます。

Julia:　What?!
　　　　何 ?!

動画 6

あなた：What is your blood pressure, Brian?
　　　　ブライアンさん、あなたの血圧は？

Brian:　My blood pressure is 145 over 90
　　　　私の血圧は、上が 145 下が 90 です。

あなた： Are you experiencing any stress now?
ストレスを感じていますか？

Brian:　 Maybe I am.
たぶん、そうです。
What is your blood pressure?
あなたの血圧は？

あなた： My blood pressure is @@over@@.
私の血圧は、上が…下が…です。
What is your blood pressure?
あなたの血圧は何ですか？

Julia:　 It is a bit low in the mornings. I wonder why?
朝は低めでだね。どうしてだろ？

あなた： Have you ever been on a diet?
ダイエットをしたことありますか？

Julia:　 I am on a diet now. Maybe that is the cause.
ダイエット中です。それが原因かしら。

Brian:　 That could be it.
そうかもね。

Lesson 11: Prescription

薬は患者の健康回復のために必要である。しかし、患者に必要な量の倍量の薬を投与したり、患者に必要な時間に薬を投与するのを忘れていたりしたら、治療の妨げになりうる。場合によっては深刻な結果につながることもある。そのために看護師は患者にどんな薬をどれだけ、そして、どんなタイミングで投与するべきか、細心の注意を払う必要がある。

1. Core Terms

1. medication　　2. painkiller　　3. tablet　　4. each　　5. meal
6. upset　　7. お腹　　8. 抗生剤　　9. 錠剤　　10. コース
11. 飲み残し

4. Core Phrases

1. お薬の説明をします。　　　　　　　2. 1回1錠、1日3回、毎食後に服用してください。
3. お薬で胃が荒れます。　　　　　　　4. 必ず食後に摂ってください。
5. こちらの抗生剤を1週間服用することになります。
6. 必ず飲み切ってください。
7. お水で飲んでください。コーヒーやジュースではなく。

7. Workout with Julia

	What	Why	When
(1)	ステロイド steroid	発疹のため for rashes	1日に数回 apply several times a day
(2)	解熱剤 fever reducer	熱を下げるため to reduce your fever	毎食後に1錠 take one pill after each meal
(3)	痛み止め painkiller	痛みを抑えるため to reduce your pain	痛いときに1錠（6時間空けること） take one pill whenever you have pain (leave six hours between doses)
(4)	睡眠導入剤 sleeping pill	寝付きやすくするため to help you fall asleep	寝る前に1錠 take one pill before going to bed
(5)	整腸剤 anti-flatulent	下痢を和らげるため to relieve your diarrhea	毎食後に2錠 take two tablets after each meal
(6)	咳止め cough medicine	咳を和らげるため to relieve your coughing	毎食後に1錠 take one pill after each meal
(7)	アレルギー用目薬 allergy eye drop	痒みを抑えるため to reduce the itching	1日3回、毎回2滴 apply two drops at a time, three times a day

8. Dialogs

Dialog 1

Nurse:　Mr. Bachman, I will explain your medication.
　　　　バックマンさん、お薬の説明をします。
Patient: OK.
　　　　はい。
Nurse:　These are painkillers.
　　　　こちらは痛み止めです。
Patient: Right.

Nurse:	Take 1 tablet, 3 times a day, after each meal.

Nurse: Take 1 tablet, 3 times a day, after each meal.
1回1錠、1日3回、毎食後に服用してください。

Patient: Can I take them (before) (meals)?
食事前に服用してもいいですか？

Nurse: They will upset your stomach.
胃が荒れます。
Be sure to take them after meals.
必ず食後に服用してください。

Patient: I'll (make) (sure).
必ずそうします。

Nurse: This is stomach medicine.
これは胃薬です。

Patient: I see.
はい。

Nurse: Take 1 tablet, 3 times a day, after each meal...same as pain killers.
1回1錠、1日3回、毎食後に服用してください…痛み止めと同じです。

Patient: OK.
分かりました。

Dialog 2

Nurse: Mr. Bachman, here are your antibiotics.
バックマンさん、抗生剤です。
Be sure to take 1 pill after breakfast only.
1回1錠を朝食後にのみ、必ず服用してください。

Patient: (Only) (once) in the morning?
朝に1回だけですか？

Nurse: That's right. You will take these antibiotics for 1 week.
そうです。この抗生剤を1週間服用することになります。

Patient: 1 week?
1週間も？

Nurse: Yes. Be sure to finish the course.
はい、そうです。必ず飲み切ってください。

Patient: No (leftovers)?
残したらだめですか？

Nurse: No leftovers.
残したらダメです。
Also, take it with water, not with coffee or juice.
また、コーヒーやジュースではなく、水で服用してください。

Patient: No (soft) (drinks)?
ソフトドリンクはだめですか？

Nurse: No soft drinks.
ソフトドリンクはだめです。

9. Listening Comprehension (巻末 Answer Sheet)

Dialog 1

Q1. What is the prescription for the painkillers?
痛み止めの処方は何ですか？
Take 1 tablet, 3 times a day, after each meal.
1回1錠、1日3回、毎食後に服用すること。

Q2.   What is the prescription for the stomach medicine?
　　　 胃薬の処方は何ですか？
　　　 Take 1 tablet, 3 times a day, after each meal. (It is the same as pain killers.)
　　　 1回1錠、1日3回、毎食後に服用すること。（痛み止めと同じである）

Dialog 2

Q1.   What is the prescription for the antibiotics?
　　　 抗生剤の処方は何ですか？
　　　 Take 1 pill after breakfast for 1 week.
　　　 朝食後に1錠を1週間服用すること。

Q2.   What should the patient take the antibiotics with?
　　　 患者は抗生剤を何と一緒に服用しなければいけませんか？
　　　 The patient should take antibiotics with water.
　　　 患者は抗生剤を水で服用しなければならない。

10. Patient Interview （5）

	箇所	症状
1		nausea／吐き気
2	joints／関節	pain／痛み 補足（動かしづらい）
3		high fever／高熱 補足（しんどい）
4	knees／膝	scrape／擦り傷 補足（自転車に乗っていてこけた）
5		blood in my phlegm／痰に血が混ざっている

Lesson 12: Common Cold

風邪は一年中引くことがある。しかし、寒い季節が近づくにつれて、件数は急激に増える。誰でものどの痛み、鼻詰まり、鼻水、咳、軽い頭痛、くしゃみ、発熱、および、軽い体の痛みを経験したことがある。風邪に対する最良の対処法は、暖かくして、しっかりと休むことだ。もちろん、水分補給もお忘れなく。

1. Core Terms

1. cold	2. symptom	3. fever	4. cough	5. flu
6. influenza	7. result	8. （熱が）出る	9. 絶え間なく	10. 食欲
11.（食事の）ひとくち		12. 鼻孔	13. 不快な	14. 支える
15. ティッシュ				

4. Core Phrases

1. 咳はいつ始まりましたか？
2. 食欲はいかがですか？
3. インフルエンザの検査をします。
4. この綿棒をお鼻に入れます。
5. 数秒間は不快な感じがします。
6. 頭の後ろを手で支えますよ。
7. 結果が出るまで３０分お待ちください。

6. Warm-up

1. capsule カプセル	2. tablet 錠剤	3. powdered medicine 粉薬
4. syrup シロップ	5. ointment 軟膏	6. eye drop 目薬
7. lozenge トローチ	8. suppository 座薬	9. compress 湿布

7. Workout with Julia

part 2

1. Take 2 (capsules), three times a day, after each meal.
2. Take 1 (tablet), once a day, before bedtime.
3. Take this (powdered) (medicine) between meals.
4. Take one spoonful of this (syrup) after each meal.
5. Apply this (ointment) several times a day.
6. Use this (eye) (drop) when it is itchy.

8. Dialogs

Dialog 1

Nurse: What seems to be the problem?
         どうされましたか？
Patient: I seem to have (caught) (a) (cold).
         風邪を引いたみたいです。
Nurse: What are the symptoms?
         症状は何ですか？
Patient: I think I am (running) (a) (fever).
         発熱しているようです。
Nurse: Are there any other symptoms?
         他に症状はありますか？
Patient: I am (constantly) (coughing).
         ずっと咳が続いています。
Nurse: When did the cough start?

咳はいつ始まりましたか？

Patient: It started last night.
昨夜からです。

Nurse: ...and how is your appetite?
で、食欲はいかがですか？

Patient: I don't feel like eating. I haven't (had) (a) (bite) since yesterday.
ありません。昨日からひとくちも食べていません。

Nurse: I see.
分かりました。

Dialog 2

Nurse: You might have the flu.
インフルエンザかもしれません。

Patient: Oh my gosh!
なんてこった！

Nurse: We will do an influenza test.
インフルエンザの検査をします。

Patient: (What) (kind) (of) test will that be?
それはどのような検査ですか？

Nurse: I will put this Q-Tip in your nostril.
この綿棒を鼻の穴に入れます。

Patient: Will it hurt?
痛いですか？

Nurse: It might feel uncomfortable for a few seconds.
数秒の間は不快に感じるかもしれません。

(moments later)
（しばらくして）

Nurse: I will support the back of your head with my hand...hold on.
手で後頭部を支えます…我慢してくださいね。

Nurse: Here you are. (handing tissue paper)
はい、どうぞ。（ティッシュを渡しながら）

Patient: Thanks.
どうも。

Nurse: We are finished. Please wait 30 minutes for the results.
はい、終わりました。結果が出るまで 30 分間待ってください。

9. Listening Comprehension （巻末 Answer Sheet）

Dialog 1

Q1.   What are the symptoms?
症状は何ですか？
The patient is running a fever and is constantly coughing.
患者は発熱をしており絶えず咳をしている。

Q2.   How is the patient's appetite?
患者の食欲はどうですか？
The patient has no appetite.
患者は食欲がない。

Dialog 2

Q1.   What kind of influenza test will the patient take?
患者が受けるインフルエンザの検査は何ですか？
The nurse will put a Q-Tip in his nostril.
看護師は彼の鼻に綿棒を入れる。

Q2.　How long should the patient wait for the result?
　　　患者は結果が出るまでどれくらい待たなければいけませんか？
　　　The patient should wait 30 minutes.
　　　患者は 30 分間待つ必要がある。

10. Vocabulary Test

1. cold　　　　2. fever　　　　3. cough　　　　4. influenza　　　5. result
6. constantly　7. appetite　　8. nostril　　　9. uncomfortable　10. support

Lesson 13: Influenza

ナースカナのワンポイントアドバイス

冬の到来と共に、インフルエンザの件数も徐々に増える。私たち看護師は、自分がインフルエンザにかからないように努めるのが重要であり。また、インフルエンザにかからないだけではなく、媒介者になり患者に伝染さないようにしなければならない。そのために、こまめに手洗いやうがい、消毒を行うこと。私たちは目に見えない敵と戦っているからこそ、細心の注意が必要である。

1. Core Terms

1. positive
2. spread
3. temperature
4. stay away
5. wear
6. nutrition
7. 病欠（病気休暇）
8. 処方する
9. 液体
10. 休む
11. 勧める
12. 消化
13. 後に

4. Core Phrases

1. 仕事に行ってはいけません。
2. 周囲の人から出来るだけ離れてください。
3. 必ずマスクを着けておいてください。
4. 必ずスポーツドリンクなどで水分補給をしてください。
5. 必ず睡眠と栄養をよく摂ってください。
6. 消化に良いものを食べてください。
7. 必ず温かくしてください。
8. 睡眠をよくとってください。

7. Workout with Julia

Part 1

	Rate of pain（数値）	Nature of pain（性質）	Movement of pain（移動）
Case 1	5	It hurts when the patient moves around. 動き回ると痛む。	It is spreading. 広がっている。
Case 2	4 (8 this morning)	The pain stops when the patient lies down and rests. 横になって休むと痛みは止まる。	No. なし。
Case 3	2 → 7	No matter what the patient does, it hurts! 何をやっても痛む。	No. なし。

Part 2

On a scale of zero to ten, how would you rate your pain?

Does anything make it better or worse?

Does the pain move anywhere?

Please rate your pain on a scale of zero to ten.

8. Dialogs

Dialog 1

Nurse: What did the doctor say?
          先生はなんと仰っていましたか？

Patient: I (tested) (positive) for influenza.
          インフルエンザ陽性反応が出ました。

Nurse: That is too bad.
          それはお気の毒ですね。

Patient: What should I do? Can I go to work?
          どうすればよいですか？仕事は行けますか？

Nurse: You may not go to work. You don't want to spread your flu to others.

仕事へ行ってはいけません。他の人にインフルエンザを伝染したくないですよね。

Patient: I see. Then, I will (ask) my boss (for) (sick) (leave).
分かりました。ならば上司に病気休暇を申請します。

Patient: When can I go back to work?
いつ復帰できますか？

Nurse: Usually, 48 hours after your temperature returns to normal.
通常ならば、体温が平熱に戻ってから 48 時間後です。

Patient: OK. How about meeting other people?
分かりました。人と会うのはどうですか？

Nurse: Try to stay away from others as much as possible.
出来るだけ他の人と距離を取ってください。

Nurse: Also, be sure to wear a mask at all times.
また、マスクをずっと着けておくように。

Dialog 2

Patient: What kind of (treatment) will I (receive)?
どのような治療を受けますか？

Nurse: We will prescribe medication.
お薬を処方します。

Patient: I see.
なるほど。

Nurse: And please be sure to take fluids such as sports drinks.
そして、スポーツドリンクのような水分を必ず摂るようにしてください。

Patient: OK.
はい。

Nurse: Also, be sure to rest well and get nutrition.
また、よく休んで栄養も摂ってください。

Patient: What kind of food is (recommended)?
どのような食べ物がお勧めですか？

Nurse: Take food that helps your digestion.
消化に良いものを食べてください。

Patient: What about (taking) (showers)?
シャワーを浴びるのはどうですか？

Nurse: You may take showers but be sure to keep warm afterwards.
シャワーを浴びてもいいですが、必ずその後は暖かくしてくださいね。

Patient: OK, I'll try.
はい、そうします。

Nurse: Finally, forget about your work and get a lot of sleep.
最後に、仕事のことは忘れて、しっかり睡眠をとってください。

Patient: That's not bad!
それも悪くないね！

9. Listening Comprehension （巻末 Answer Sheet）

Dialog 1

Q1. What was the result of the test?
検査結果はどうでしたか？
The result of the test was positive.
検査の結果は陽性であった。

Q2. When can the patient go back to work?
患者はいつ仕事に戻れますか？
The patient can go back to work 48 hours after his temperature returns to normal.

患者は体温が平熱に戻ってから 48 時間後に仕事に復帰してもよい。

Dialog 2

Q1. What kind of drinks are recommended?
どんな飲み物が勧められていますか？

Sports drinks are recommended.
スポーツ飲料が勧められている。

Q2. What kind of food is recommended?
どんな食べ物が勧められていますか？

Food that helps digestion is recommended.
消化に良い食べ物が勧められている。

10. Patient Interview （6）

	箇所	症状
1	頭／head	ふらふらする、吐き気／light headed, queasy
2		咳／cough 補足（3週間前から、今は血が混じっている）
3	（喉）/ (throat)	飲み込む時に痛む、熱っぽい／ pain when swallowing, feverish
4		下痢／diarrhea 補足（最近仕事のストレスが溜まっている）
5	お腹／stomach	お腹が張っている、便意がない／ bloated, no bowel movement

Lesson 14: External Injury

ナースカナのワンポイントアドバイス

外傷は事故や転倒などによって起こる。擦り傷などの軽微なものかもしれない。しかし、場合によっては、命に関わることもある。痛みや出血により、患者はパニックに陥ることもある。血を見ただけで、気を失う場合もある。そんなときでも、慌てずに！必要な処置が素早く受けられるように、冷静な対応が求められる。

1. Core Terms

1. fall
2. knee
3. scrape
4. bleed
5. disinfect
6. gauze
7. すべる
8. 舗道
9. 傷口（打ち身）
10. 骨
11. 患部
12. チクっとする
13. 取る

4. Core Phrases

1. どうされたんですか？
2. 膝を見ましょう。
3. 傷口をきれいにします。
4. 先生に診てもらいます。
5. 患部を消毒します。
6. 少しチクッとします。
7. ガーゼを取らないでください。

6. Warm-up

1. 首
2. 額
3. 肩
4. 胸
5. お腹
6. 上腕
7. 肘
8. 前腕部
9. 手首
10. 手のひら
11. 腿
12. 膝
13. 脛
14. ふくらはぎ
15. 足首
16. 背中
17. 背骨

7. Workout with Julia

1. This is the neck.
2. This is the temple.
3. This is the shoulder.
4. This is the chest.
5. This is the stomach.
6. This is the upper arm.
7. This is the elbow.
8. This is the forearm.
9. This is the wrist.
10. This is the palm.
11. This is the thigh.
12. This is the knee.
13. This is the shin.
14. This is the calf.
15. This is the ankle.
16. This is the back.
17. This is the spine.

8. Dialogs

Dialog 1

Nurse: What seems to be the problem?
どうなさいましたか？

Patient: I (fell) and (hurt) my (knee).
こけて膝を怪我しました。

Nurse: How did it happen?
どうしてですか？

Patient: My bicycle slipped and I (hit) my knee (on) the pavement.
自転車がすべって、舗道に膝を打ち付けました。

Nurse: Did you hit your head or any other part of your body?
頭か体のほかの部分は打ちましたか？

Patient: I didn't hit my head...but I (scraped) my hand.
頭は打っていません…が、手を擦りむきました。

Nurse: I see. First, let's take a look at your knee.
なるほど。まずは、膝を見ましょう。

Patient: Awww! It's (bleeding)!

うわぁ！血が出ている！
Nurse: Don't worry, I will clean the bruise and have the doctor check it.
心配しないでください。傷口をきれいにして先生に診てもらいましょう。

Dialog 2
Nurse: The x-ray shows there were no broken bones.
レントゲンの結果、骨折はありませんでした。
Patient: Oh, that is a (relief)!
あぁ、それは安心しました！
Nurse: So, I will disinfect the site.
では、患部を消毒します。
Patient: Will it hurt?
痛みますか？
Nurse: It may sting a little but you will be OK.
少ししみますが、大丈夫ですよ。
(moments later)
（しばらくして）
Patient: Can I take a shower today?
今日はシャワーを浴びてもいいですか？
Nurse: No. Please wait until tomorrow.
ダメです。明日まで待ってください。
Patient: Do I (return) tomorrow?
明日も来院しなくてはなりませんか？
Nurse: Yes. I will check your bruise again.
はい。傷口を再度見ます。
Nurse: Until then, do not remove the gauze.
それまではガーゼを外さないでくださいね。

9. Listening Comprehension （巻末 Answer Sheet）

Dialog 1
Q1.   How did the patient hurt his knee?
患者はどのようにして膝を痛めたのですか？
His bicycle slipped and he hit his knee on the pavement.
彼の自転車が滑って膝を舗道にぶつけた。
Q2.   What will the nurse do before the doctor checks?
医師の診察の前に看護師は何をしますか？
The nurse will clean the bruise.
看護師は傷口をきれいにします。

Dialog 2
Q1.   What is the result of the x-ray?
X線の結果は何ですか？
There were no broken bones.
骨折はなかった。
Q2.   When can the patient take a shower?
患者はいつシャワーを浴びられますか？
The patient can take a shower tomorrow.
患者は明日シャワーを浴びることができる。

10. Vocabulary Test
1. fall   2. knee   3. scrape   4. bleed   5. disinfect
6. gauze   7. bruise   8. bone   9. site   10. sting

Lesson 15: Loss of Appetite

ナースカナのワンポイントアドバイス

食べることは私たちの健康において中心的な役割を果たしている。したがって食欲不振は大きな問題になりうる。原因を探り、医師や栄養士と相談することも看護師の役割のひとつといえる。患者にとって最もふさわしい食べ物は何かを考えること。食感や、温度、一口のサイズ、トレイやスプーンの選択など、工夫できることはある。

1. Core Terms

1. appetite
2. nausea
3. stress
4. tough
5. pressure
6. examine
7. 胸焼け
8. 血液サンプル
9. 尿サンプル
10. 胃カメラ
11. 麻酔スプレー

4. Core Phrases

1. いつからですか？
2. 吐き気はありますか？
3. 何か食べられるものはありますか？
4. 最近ストレスをお感じになっていますか？
5. いくつかの検査をします。
6. 血液と尿の採取をします。
7. レントゲンとCTスキャンもします。
8. 胃カメラで検査をします。

7. Workout with Julia

	What	Why	When
(1)	acid reducing drug 胃酸抑制剤	treat heartburn 胸焼け治療のため	(take one pill once a day) after breakfast (1日1錠)朝食後
(2)	nitrate 舌下剤	for chest pains 胸の痛みのため	when you have chest pains 胸の痛みがある時
(3)	anti-allergy medicine 抗アレルギー薬	relive hay fever 花粉症を和らげるため	(take one pill twice a day) after breakfast and before sleeping (1錠ずつ1日2回)朝食後と就寝前
(4)	inhaler 吸入器	to make it easy to breathe 呼吸を楽にするため	(inhale) when you have trouble breathing 呼吸がしづらい時に(吸入する)
(5)	burn cream やけど軟膏	to decrease burn pain 火傷の痛みを和らげるため	(apply once a day) after showering (and cover with gauze) (1日1回)シャワー後に(塗った後にガーゼで覆う)
(6)	compress 湿布	to decrease back pain 腰痛を和らげるため	(apply) when you have pain 痛みがある時に(貼る)
(7)	laxative 下剤	to treat constipation 便秘の治療のため	(apply 10 drops into a glass of water and drink) before going to sleep (コップ1杯の水に10滴たらして)寝る前に(飲む)

8. Dialogs

Dialog 1

Nurse: What seems to be the problem?
どうなさいましたか？

Patient: I seem to have (lost) my (appetite).
食欲がありません。

Nurse: Since when?
いつからですか？

Patient: For about (the) (past) (two) (weeks).
約 2 週間前からです。

Nurse: Do you have any nausea?
吐き気はありますか？

Patient: I do not have any nausea but I have (heartburn).
吐き気はありませんが、胸焼けはあります。

Nurse: Is there anything that you can eat?
何か食べれるものはありますか？

Patient: I can eat (bananas).
バナナを食べれます。

Nurse: Are you experiencing any stress now?
今ストレスを感じていますか？

Patient: I am having a (tough) (time) at work. I feel a lot of (pressure).
仕事が大変です。プレッシャーをたくさん感じています。

Dialog 2

Nurse: Mr. Bachman, we will do some tests.
バックマンさん、検査をいくつかします。

Patient: (What) (kind) (of) tests will you do?
どのような検査をするのですか？

Nurse: Today, we will take a blood sample and urine sample.
今日は、血液サンプルと尿サンプルを採取します。

Patient: I see.
分かりました。

Nurse: We will also take an x-ray and a CT scan.
またレントゲンと CT スキャンも撮ります。

Patient: Will that be all?
それで全てですか？

Nurse: There is one more. Next week, we will examine with an endoscope.
もう一つあります。来週、エンドスコープ（胃カメラ）で検査をします。

Patient: What is that?
それは何ですか？

Nurse: It is a camera to look inside your stomach.
あなたの胃の中を診るためのカメラです。

Patient: Ugh. (Sounds) (tough).
うわぁ。辛そう。

Nurse: It is, but we will use some anesthetic spray.
確かにそうですが、麻酔スプレーを使いますよ。

9. Listening Comprehension （巻末 Answer Sheet）

Dialog 1

Q1.   When did the patient lose his appetite?
いつ患者は食欲をなくしましたか？
The patient lost his appetite two weeks ago.
患者は 2 週間前に食欲をなくした。

Q2.   Why is the patient experiencing stress?
なぜ患者はストレスを感じているのですか？
The patient is having a tough time at work. He feels a lot of pressure.
患者は仕事が大変である。多くのプレッシャーを感じている。

Dialog 2

Q1. What kind of samples will be collected?
何のサンプルが採取されますか？

A blood sample and urine sample will be collected.
血液と尿が採取される。

Q2. What is an endoscope?
エンドスコープ（胃カメラ）とは何ですか？

It is a camera to look inside the stomach.
胃の中を診るためのカメラです。

10. Patient Interview（7）

	箇所	症状
1		息切れと呼吸時にゼーゼーする。／ shortness of breath and wheezing sound when she breathes
2	頭／ head	ボーっとする。／ dazed 補足（梯子から落ちて頭を打った。）
3	関節と頭／ joints and head	発熱と痛み／ running a fever, headache, and joints are aching
4	鼻腔／ sinus	完全な鼻詰まり、濃痰、頭が重い／ totally blocked, green phlegm, and head feels heavy
5	腕や足／ arms and legs	あざ／ bruises

QRコードで動画が見られる!

看護英語ワークブック

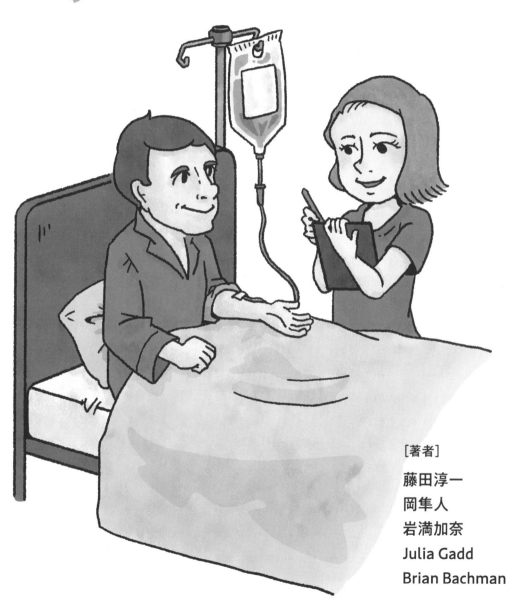

[著者]

藤田淳一
岡隼人
岩満加奈
Julia Gadd
Brian Bachman

Kinpodo

はじめに

　看護師を目指している皆さん、こんにちは！まずは、看護師を目指してくださり、わたしはとても嬉しく思っています。こんなに素晴らしい仕事は他にないと思うぐらい、看護師の仕事は楽しいです。今は勉強が大変な時期かもしれませんが、看護師になりたいと思った気持ちをいつまでも忘れず、ステキな看護師になってくださいね。

　さて、日々、授業や実習に奮闘しているなかで、英語も学ばなければならないと思うと、気が重いかもしれませんね。わたしも学生のころはそうでした。しかし、苦痛や不安を抱えた外国の患者さんに出会う場面は多々あります。この本では難しい専門用語は使わず、患者さんを知ることができるフレーズがたくさんでてきます。一つでも身につけて、看護の場面で活かせたら、看護師として自信になりますよね。世界も広がります。みなさんが今後、看護師として活躍されるのを楽しみにしています。

2021年2月

看護師　岩満加奈

　大学や専門学校ではどのような英語を勉強すればよいだろうか。例えば大学に通う学生にとって必要な英語は個人個人で異なります。就活が始まるまでにTOEICの点数を上げる、小説を原書で読めるようにする、人前で簡単な英語プレゼンテーションが出来るようになるなど様々です。

　では、看護師を目指している学生はどうでしょうか。TOEIC、英語の小説、プレゼンテーションも良いが、まずは仕事に必要不可欠な英語を身に着けることが必要ではないでしょうか。その英語とは、外国人患者が来院したときに対応できる英語です。患者は外国人であっても医療に関しては素人です。難しい専門用語は不要です。また、症状や不安を抱えて来院しています。複雑な構文や凝った表現も不要です。求められているのは、患者に通じる英語を必要な場面で的確に使う能力です。外国人患者と意思疎通が出来て安心して治療を受ければ、今までに感じたことがない語学に対する自信が湧いてきます。本テキストでは、100本以上の動画を視聴しながらワークブック形式で無理なく必要な看護英語を身に着けることができます。

　本書では、スマートフォンでQRコードを読み取って動画を視聴します。それにより、Wi-Fi環境さえあれば、いつ、どこでも看護英語の勉強をすることができます。また、すべての動画にPCからアクセスできるようURLも用意しています。LL教室やPC教室などでの授業、またより大きい画面で視聴したい方に使っていただければと思います。

2021年2月

著者代表　藤田淳一

【著者紹介】

- 藤田淳一（ふじた　じゅんいち）　大阪歯科大学英語教室
- 岡隼人（おか　はやと）　大阪歯科大学英語教室
- 岩満加奈（いわみつ　かな）　看護師
- Julia Gadd（ジュリア　ガッド）　英語講師
- Brian Bachman（ブライアン　バックマン）　英語講師

撮影協力：医療法人　秀裕会　かんやまクリニック
Special thanks to Dr. Hirokazu Akashi and Dr. Yoshihiro Yoshikawa
for their helpful advice and support.

Contents

別冊：解答集

本書の使い方

動画へのアクセス
スマートフォンにQRコードリーダーなどのアプリが事前にインストールされているか確認してください。スマートフォンでテキスト内に印刷されているQRコードを読み取ります。パスワード（2021）を入力していただきますと、そのレッスンの動画がまとめて表示されます。必要な動画を選んで再生してください。以下のURLにテキスト内のすべての動画があります。
▶ https://vimeo.com/showcase/kangoallvideos

ナースカナのワンポイントアドバイス
ナースカナが看護師として日頃心掛けていることを英語でアドバイスしています。レッスン前に軽く読んで頭を「英語モード」に切り替えましょう。

1　Core Terms
各レッスンのテーマに関連する用語です。これらの用語を英語及び日本語に訳して空所に書き込みます。授業では、学生同士でペアを組みます。片方の学生は、テキストを見ながら各用語を読み上げます。もう一方の学生は、それに対して（テキストを見ず）素早く英語又は日本語に訳します。この練習方法をQuick Responseと呼びます。英単語を目ではなく、耳で覚える練習です。

2　Brian's Pronunciation Practice（動画付き）
Core Termsで取り上げられた単語をブライアン先生が発音します。動画を見ながら彼に続いて発音の練習をしましょう。

3　Pronunciation Tips（動画付き）
日本人が特に苦手としている発音に焦点を当て、ブライアン先生が丁寧に発音してくれています。動画を見て、下線部の発音に注意しながら、先生に続いてリピートしましょう。

4　Core Phrases
各レッスンのテーマに関連するフレーズです。Core Termsを含んでいます。きっちりと日本語に訳しましょう。ここでは看護師が使うであろう英語のフレーズを習得しましょう。

5　Quick Response（動画付き）
上記4のフレーズでQuick Responseの練習をします。動画を見ながらナースカナの日本語に対する英訳を瞬時に言います。今までの英語の勉強は文字を見て覚えてきました。しかし、実

際に外国人患者の対応をするときは、文字を当てにすることはできません。相手が発した英語を聞いて即座に反応する必要があります。そこで通訳者の養成教育によく用いられるQuick Responseの練習をします。動画で読み上げられた日本語を聞いて即座に英語に訳す練習です。ポイントは動画の音声に対して即座に反応することです。

6   Warm-up（動画付きの場合あり）

Warm-upとは準備のことです。次のWorkout with Juliaに登場する単語やフレーズの解説を主にします。このWarm-upをすることで、Workout with Juliaの聞き取りや発話がしやすくなります。

7   Workout with Julia（動画付き）

Warm-upで学んだことをここで実践してみましょう。

8   Dialogs（動画付き）

外国人患者の対応で起こりうる場面を対話形式の動画にしています。まず動画を見て概要を理解してください。その後、再び動画を見ながらDialogs内の空欄を埋めます。空欄になっているのは外国人患者の返答として予測されるフレーズです。しっかりと聞き取れるようにしましょう。

9   Listening Comprehension

Dialogsの対話文の理解を深めるための練習です。8の動画をもう一度見て、巻末にある内容に関する質問に答えます。その際、テキスト中の対話文は見ずに動画の視聴のみで解きます。センテンス（主語＋動詞）の形で答えるように心がけてください。他の学習者とペアを組み、読み上げられた質問に対して口頭で答えるとより高度な練習が可能です。

10 Vocabulary Test / Patient Interview Practice（動画付きの場合あり）

Vocabulary Test（巻末のAnswer Sheet裏面）

レッスンの単語が身についているかを確認するため、単語テストが用意されています。

Patient Interview Practice（巻末のAnswer Sheet裏面）

本編では掲載しきれなかった様々な状況や症状などを問診形式で聞き取る練習をしましょう。

Lesson 1
Reception
受付

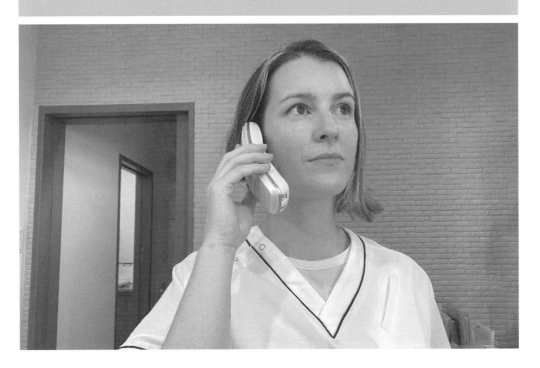

ナースカナのワンポイントアドバイス

Nurses do not appear at the reception so often. However, whenever you do, keep in mind that patients have anxiety. It is important to relieve this anxiety with sincere and careful interaction. Assessing the symptoms and then efficiently directing the patient to the proper clinic is important.

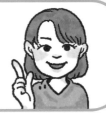

1 Core Terms
次の語を英語の場合は日本語に、日本語の場合は英語に直しなさい。

1. 看護師

2. 予約

3. 問題（p）

4. ウェブサイト

5. 問題（t）

6. 待つ

7. seem to be ～

8. stomach pains

9. right now

10. health insurance

11. fill out

12. How long ～ ?

2 Brian's Pronunciation Practice
動画の音声に続いてリピートしなさい。

3 Pronunciation Tips
動画の音声に続いて単語の発音練習をしなさい。

[s / th の発音] 1. nurse   2. website   3. sore   4. throat   5. health

4 Core Phrases
次の英文を和訳しなさい。

1. What seems to be the problem?

2. May I have your name?

3. Do you have health insurance?

4. Please fill out this form.

5. Let me know if you have any trouble with it.

6. This way please.

7. Please sit here.

8. You may go in now.

5 Quick Response
動画を見て日本語に対する英訳を瞬時に口頭で言いなさい。
瞬発力が大事です！

6 Warm-up
道案内をする時は命令文を使います。
以下の説明を読んで使い方を確認しましょう。

真っすぐ進みなさい。 →　Go straight. / Walk straight.
右に曲がりなさい、左に曲がりなさい → Turn right. / Turn left.

しかし、Go straight. Turn left. Go straight. Turn right.... では逆に分かりにくい説明になります。また単調で聞きづらいかもしれません。このように少し情報をプラスすればより分かりやすい説明になります。

Go straight + one block.	1ブロック進みなさい。（距離）
Go straight + to the convenience store.	コンビニまで進みなさい。（目的地）
Go straight + past the coffee shop.	喫茶店を通り過ぎて進みなさい。（途中の目印）
Turn right + at the corner.	角で右に曲がりなさい。（位置）

巻末にWarm-upのリスニング問題があります。

7 Workout with Julia
動画の地図を見ながら、ナースジュリアになったつもりで
患者に対して口頭で説明しなさい。約30秒で説明すること。

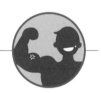

1. Hello, I am at the station. Could you give me directions?

2. Hi, I seem to be lost. I am walking by a river.

3. After the treatment, I have to go to Kinpodo. How do I get there?

8 Dialogs
動画を見て次の空欄を埋めなさい。

Dialog 1:（お腹が痛いんですけど…）
Nurse:　もしもし。かんやまクリニックです。
Patient:　Hello. I don't have an (　　　　　　　).
Nurse:　What seems to be the problem?
Patient:　I have (　　　　　　)(　　　　　　　).

Nurse: Is this your first visit to this clinic?

Patient: Yes, it is.

Nurse: Why don't you come over right now?

Patient: (   )(   )(   )

          (   )(   )?

Nurse: We have a map on our website.

Patient: OK. (   )(   )(   ) it.

Dialog 2: (こちらに記入してください)

Patient: Hello. I just called (   )(   )

          (   )....

Nurse: Oh, yes. May I have your name?

Patient: My name is Brian Bachman.

Nurse: Mr. Bachman, do you have health insurance?

Patient: (   )(   ) my Kokuminhoken card.

Nurse: Please fill out this form.

Patient: OK.

Nurse: Let me know if you have any trouble with it.

Dialog 3: (バックマンさん、どうぞ！)

Nurse: Mr. Bachman?

Patient: Yes.

Nurse: This way please.

Nurse: Please sit here.

Patient: (   )(   ) will I have to

          (   )?

Nurse: Your name will be called next.

Patient: OK. Thank you.

(moments later)

Nurse: Mr. Bachman. You may go in now.

 Listening Comprehension
「8」Dialogs の動画をもう一度見て巻末の Answer Sheet にある問題を
解きなさい。

Lesson 2
Patient Interview
問診

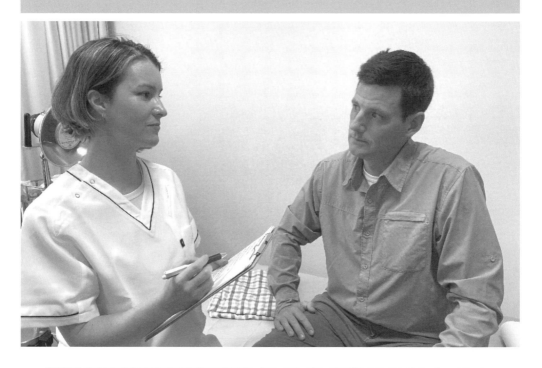

ナースカナのワンポイントアドバイス

Information concerning the patient is obtained through verbal communication. Keep in mind that non-verbal signs such as facial expressions, complexion, and how their voice sounds can tell you a lot about their condition. Show your dedicated attention in listening to the patient's complaints. This will make it easier for them to open up. Also, don't forget to respect their privacy.

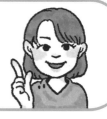

1 Core Terms
次の語を英語の場合は日本語に、日本語の場合は英語に直しなさい。

1. もう一度（a）　2. 病気（i）　3. 病院　4. 前に（b）

5. ここ最近（c）　6. アレルギー　7. serious　8. pneumonia

9. tendon　10. operation　11. surgery　12. medication

13. symptom　14. nausea　15. vomit（動詞）

2 Brian's Pronunciation Practice
動画の音声に続いてリピートしなさい。

3 Pronunciation Tips
動画の音声に続いて単語の発音練習をしなさい。

[黙字] 1. p̲nemonia　　2. k̲nee　　3. musc̲le　　4. sig̲n　　5. w̲rist

4 Core Phrases
次の英文を和訳しなさい。

1. Have you had any serious illness before?

2. Have you ever had any operations before?

3. Are you taking any medications currently?

4. Do you have any allergies?

5. Where does it particularly hurt?

6. When did the pain start?

7. Do you have any other symptoms?

5 Quick Response
動画を見て日本語に対する英訳を瞬時に口頭で言いなさい。
瞬発力が大事です！

Warm-up

動画を見てブライアン先生に続いてリピートしなさい。
次にもう一度動画を見てブライアン先生の言った英単語を和訳して
下の表を埋めなさい。

英語	日本語
notepad	
three color ballpoint pen	
ruler	
scissors	
surgical tape	
tourniquet	
watch	
hand sanitizer	
medical penlight	
personal seal	
alcohol swab	
calculator	
bandage	

Workout with Julia

動画を見てナースジュリアの質問（What's this? /
これは何ですか？）に英語の文（This is ~ / これは～です。）
で答えなさい。

8 Dialogs

動画を見て次の空欄を埋めなさい。

Dialog 1:（今までに手術を受けたことはありますか？）

Nurse:　May I have your name again?

Patient: My name is Brian Bachman.

Nurse:　Have you had any serious illnesses before?

Patient: I was (　　　　　　　) (　　　　　　　) (　　　　　　　) with
　　　　 (　　　　　　　) last year.

Nurse:　Have you ever had any operations before?

Patient: I (　　　　　　　) my (　　　　　　　) and (　　　　　　　)
　　　　 (　　　　　　　) a few years ago.

Nurse:　Are you taking any medications currently?

Patient: No, I am not.

Nurse:　Do you have any allergies?

Patient: Yes, I am (　　　　　　　) (　　　　　　　) peanuts.

Dialog 2:（特にどこが痛みますか？）

Nurse:　What seems to be the problem?

Patient: I am having (　　　　　　　) (　　　　　　　).

Nurse:　Where does it particularly hurt?

Patient: The (　　　　　　　) (　　　　　　　) (　　　　　　　) hurts.

Nurse:　When did the pain start?

Patient: It started (　　　　　　　) (　　　　　　　).

Nurse:　Do you have any other symptoms?

Patient: I have (　　　　　　　) and I (　　　　　　　) several times.

9 Listening Comprehension

「8」Dialogsの動画をもう一度見て巻末のAnswer Sheetにある問題を
解きなさい。

10 Vocabulary Test

巻末のAnswer Sheetの裏面にある単語テストを受けなさい。

Lesson 3
Body Temperature and Pulse
体温・脈拍測定

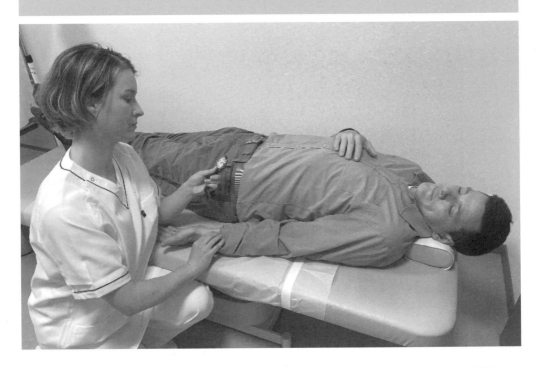

ナースカナのワンポイントアドバイス

Measuring the pulse means there will be direct contact with the patient's body surface. Make sure that you do not have cold hands. You would not want to surprise the patient. Before asking them to roll up their sleeve, show consideration for patient privacy by offering to close the curtain. Be sure to explain in advance, what procedure you will be doing. This will help avoid unnecessary tension. When taking temperatures, don't forget to ask what their normal temperature is.

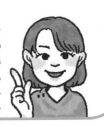

1 Core Terms
次の語を英語の場合は日本語に、日本語の場合は英語に直しなさい。

1. 生年月日（3語） 2. カーテン   3. プライバシー 4. 手首   5. 分

6. 通常（n）   7. temperature 8. thermometer 9. Fahrenheit 10. Celsius

11. rate   12. beat   13. per   14. a bit   15. nervous

2 Brian's Pronunciation Practice
動画の音声に続いてリピートしなさい。

3 Pronunciation Tips
動画の音声に続いて単語の発音練習をしなさい。

[ə] 1. curtain 2. hurt 3. nurse 4. birth 5. nervous

4 Core Phrases
次の英文を和訳しなさい。

1. May I have your date of birth?

2. I am going to take your temperature.

3. May I have the thermometer, please?

4. What is your normal temperature?

5. Please take off your shoes and lie down.

6. Shall I pull the curtain?

7. May I have your wrist?

8. Are you nervous?

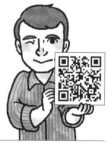

5 Quick Response
動画を見て日本語に対する英訳を瞬時に口頭で言いなさい。
瞬発力が大事です！

6 Warm-up
次の英文を和訳しなさい。

1. Are you under a physician's care now?　　※under 〜 = 〜の下

2. Have you ever been hospitalized?　　※hospitalize = 入院させる

3. Have you ever had a major operation?　　　※major = 主要な、大きな

4. Are you taking any medication now?

5. Are you on any special diet?

6. Do you use tobacco?

7. Do you drink alcohol?

 Workout with Julia
動画の中の2つのケースに関する答えを聴き取って、
日本語で簡潔に書きなさい。

	Case 1	Case 2
1. Are you under a physician's care now?		
2. Have you ever been hospitalized?		
3. Have you ever had a major operation?		
4. Are you taking any medication now?		
5. Are you on any special diet?		
6. Do you use tobacco?		
7. Do you drink alcohol?		

 Dialogs
動画を見て次の空欄を埋めなさい。

Dialog 1:（あなたの体温は 36.9 度です）
Nurse:　May I have your name?
Patient: My name is Brian Bachman.
Nurse:　May I have your date of birth?

Patient: My birthday is (   ) (   ),
(   ).

Nurse: OK.

Nurse: I am going to take your temperature under your arm now.

Nurse: May I have the thermometer, please?

Nurse: Thank you. Your temperature is 36.9.

Patient: OK.

Nurse: What is your normal temperature?

Patient: It is around (   ) (   ) Fahrenheit...which is
about (   ) (   ).

Nurse: I see. OK, we are finished, thank you.

Patient: Thanks.

Dialog 2: (脈拍 100 回／分は速いですか？)

Nurse: Please take off your shoes and lie down.

Nurse: Shall I pull the curtain for privacy?

Patient: Yes, please.

Nurse: Now I am going to take your pulse.

Patient: OK.

Nurse: May I have your wrist?

Patient: Here.

Nurse: I am going to feel your pulse now...Just relax.

(after one minute)

Nurse: Your pulse rate is 100 beats per minute.

Patient: Is that OK?

Nurse: It is a bit fast. Are you nervous?

Patient: (   ), (   ) (   ).

Nurse: Between 60 and 100 is normal for an adult.

Patient: Oh, good. Thank you.

9 Listening Comprehension

「8」Dialogs の動画をもう一度見て巻末の Answer Sheet にある問題を
解きなさい。

10 Patient Interview Practice

巻末の Answer Sheet の裏面にある問題を解きなさい。

Lesson 4
Blood Pressure
血圧測定

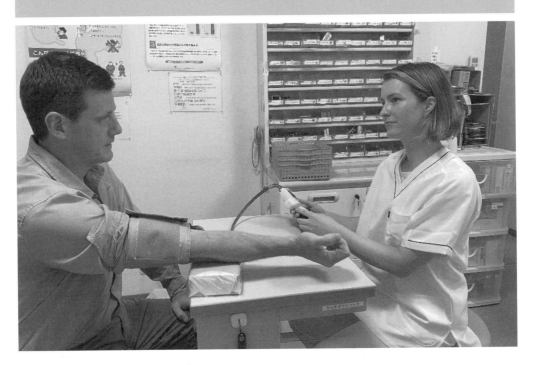

ナースカナのワンポイントアドバイス

Doing exercise, taking baths, and having meals affect blood pressure. It is necessary to do the measurements when the body is at rest. So, make sure by checking on this point before starting the procedure. If not, you will end up doing it once again...just like in the dialog video of this lesson. Once in a while, there are patients whose blood pressure starts rising just by looking at a nurse in uniform!

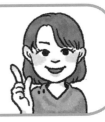

1 Core Terms
次の語を英語の場合は日本語に、日本語の場合は英語に直しなさい。

1. 測る(t)	2. テーブル	3. 秒
4. 圧迫する(s)	5. 外す(r)	6. （組んだ足などを）戻す
7. blood pressure	8. cuff	9. pump up
10. prefer	11. usually	12. for a while

2 Brian's Pronunciation Practice
動画の音声に続いてリピートしなさい。

3 Pronunciation Tips
動画の音声に続いて単語の発音練習をしなさい。

[ʃ] 1. pressure　　2. sure　　3. insurance　　4. operation　　5. special

4 Core Phrases
次の英文を和訳しなさい。

1. I am going to take your blood pressure.

2. Please put your arm on the table.

3. I am going to place this cuff around your arm.

4. I am going to pump up the cuff.

5. It will squeeze your arm just a little bit.

6. I will remove this cuff.

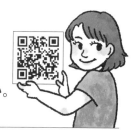

5 Quick Response
動画を見て日本語に対する英訳を瞬時に口頭で言いなさい。
瞬発力が大事です！

6 Warm-up
次の文は患者に伝える指示です。各文を和訳しなさい。

▶手
1. Show me your palm.

2. Show me the back of your hand.

▶腕

3. Straighten your arm.

4. Bend your arm.

5. Raise your arm.

6. Put down your arm.

▶足

7. Straighten your leg.（寝ている状態）

8. Bend your knees.（寝ている状態）

▶全身

9. Please sit down.

10. Lie down with you head this way.（寝ている状態）

11. Please lie down facing the wall.（寝ている状態）

12. Please relax.（寝ている状態）

 Workout with Julia
ナースジュリアと患者のやり取りを動画で見なさい。
次に、ナースジュリアに代わって先程と同じ指示を英語で
出しなさい。

 Dialogs
動画を見て次の空欄を埋めなさい。

Dialog 1:（血圧を測りますね！）

Nurse: I am going to take your blood pressure.

Patient: OK.

Nurse: Please put your arm on the table.

Patient: Sure.

Nurse: I am going to place this cuff around your arm.

Nurse: Now, I am going to pump up the cuff.

Nurse: It will squeeze your arm just a little bit.

But it will only be for a few seconds.

Patient: (   ) (   ).

Nurse: 120 over 82.

Patient: (   ) (   ) (   ).

Nurse: I will remove this cuff.

Dialog 2:（測り直し！）

Nurse: Could you uncross your legs, please?

Patient: Oh, OK.

Nurse: Which arm do you prefer?

Patient: Umm... (   ) (   ) (   ).

Nurse: May I push up your sleeve?

Patient: Sure.

Nurse: 140 over 95.

Patient: What?!

Nurse: Is it usually this high?

Patient: It seems (   ) (   ) (   ).

Nurse: Did you do anything to raise your blood pressure?

Patient: I just (   ) (   ) (   ) to this room.

Nurse: OK, let's try it again 30 minutes later.

Nurse: Please keep still for a while.

Patient: Sure.

9 Listening Comprehension

「8」Dialogs の動画をもう一度見て巻末の Answer Sheet にある問題を解きなさい。

10 Vocabulary Test

巻末の Answer Sheet の裏面にある単語テストを受けなさい。

Lesson 5
Blood and Urine Sampling
採血・採尿

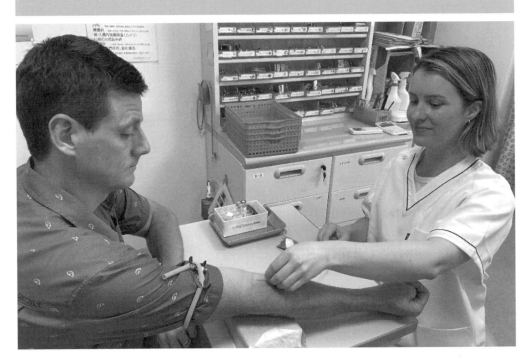

ナースカナのワンポイントアドバイス

Taking blood samples can be a painful experience for the patient. That is why it is important to get it done swiftly in one try. Remember, practice makes perfect. Collecting samples of body fluid is vital in obtaining information about the patient's condition. So, extra care is necessary in the handling and management of these samples. In the case of urine samples, the collecting is done by the patient themselves. Be sure they know exactly how to do it.

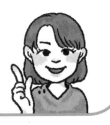

---

1 Core Terms
次の語を英語の場合は日本語に、日本語の場合は英語に直しなさい。

---

1. 枕（腕置き）　2. 真っ直ぐに　3. 拳　　4. 親指　　5. 見える状態

6. 針　　　7. vein　　8. disinfect　9. site　　10. slight

11. numbness　12. nausea　　13. urine　　14. container　15. remaining

Brian's Pronunciation Practice
動画の音声に続いてリピートしなさい。

 Pronunciation Tips
動画の音声に続いて単語の発音練習をしなさい。

［ài］ 1. site   2. slight   3. cry   4. time   5. privacy

4 **Core Phrases**
次の英文を和訳しなさい。

1. Put your arm on this pillow, please.

2. Hold your arm out straight.

3. Make a fist with your thumb inside.

4. I will disinfect the site.

5. I am going to put the needle in now.

6. You will feel a slight pain.

7. I am going to take the needle out now.

8. Press on this to stop the bleeding.

 Quick Response
動画を見て日本語に対する英訳を瞬時に口頭で言いなさい。
瞬発力が大事です！

6 Warm-up
様々な痛みの種類を答え方のパターンに当てはめて英語で言えるようにしなさい。

痛みの種類

痛みの種類の訊き方はWhat kind of pain is it?　さえ覚えていれば十分です。
答え方としては、以下の二通りが主に考えられます。

● It's a ~ pain.

● I have a ~ pain.

様々な痛みの種類についてはP.74を参照。

7 Workout with Julia
動画を見て、各患者の痛みの種類と場所を英語もしくは
日本語で書きなさい。

	痛みの種類	痛みの場所
1		
2		
3		
4		
5		
6		
7		
8		
9		
10		
11		
12		
13		

8 Dialogs
動画を見て次の空欄を埋めなさい。

Dialog 1:（血液を採ります）

Nurse:　Mr. Bachman, I need to take some blood for a test.

Patient: OK.

Nurse:　Put your arm on this pillow, please.

Patient: Sure.

Nurse:　Hold your arm out straight.

Patient: (　　　　　　　)(　　　　　　　)?

Nurse:　Yes. I will wrap this tourniquet around your arm.

Nurse: Make a fist with your thumb inside to make your veins visible.

Patient: OK.

Nurse: I will disinfect the site. It will feel a bit cold.

Nurse: I am going to put the needle in now.

Patient: (   )(   )(   )?

Nurse: You will feel a slight pain.

Nurse: Do you feel any numbness or nausea?

Patient: No, I don't.

Nurse: I am going to take the needle out now.

Nurse: OK. We are finished.

Patient: Pheew!

Nurse: Press on this to stop the bleeding.

Dialog 2:（どこまで入れるのですか？）

Nurse: We need to collect a urine sample, OK?

Patient: Sure.

Nurse: Here is the container.

Patient: (   )(   )(   )
         (   )(   )?

Nurse: First, pass a small amount of urine into the toilet.

Patient: I'll try.

Nurse: Then start collecting your urine into the container.

Patient: (   )(   )(   )
         (   )(   ) ?

Nurse: Fill up to the line.

Patient: I see.

Nurse: After collecting the sample, pass the remaining urine into the toilet.

Patient: OK.

Nurse: Also, do not touch the inside of the container.

9 Listening Comprehension

「8」Dialogs の動画をもう一度見て巻末の Answer Sheet にある問題を
解きなさい。

10 Patient Interview Practice

巻末の Answer Sheet の裏面にある問題を解きなさい。

英会話コーナー 1

 英会話上達のコツ

> **コツ ❶** 質問に対して単語のみではなく、主語・動詞をつけて文で答えるように心がける。

例　**質問**　What is your favorite fruit?
　　　　　好きな果物は何ですか？

　　回答　Strawberry (Strawberries). ✕
　　　　　いちご。

　　　　　My favorite fruit is strawberry (strawberries).　○
　　　　　わたしの好きな果物はいちごです。

次の各質問に対する返事を完成させよう。（質問の太字が回答の主語・動詞に使われる）

●**質問**

What is your name?
名前は？

Where do you live?
どこに住んでいるか？

How do you get to school?
通学方法は？

What is your favorite food?
好きな食べ物は？

What is your favorite topping?
好きな（ピザ）トッピングは？

What is your hobby?
趣味は？

●**回答**

My name is ＿＿＿＿＿＿＿＿＿＿＿＿＿＿

I live in ＿＿＿＿＿＿＿＿＿＿＿＿＿＿＿

I get to school by ＿＿＿＿＿＿＿＿＿＿

My favorite food is ＿＿＿＿＿＿＿＿＿

My favorite topping is ＿＿＿＿＿＿＿＿

My hobby is ＿＿＿＿＿＿＿＿＿＿＿＿＿

コツ**2**　こちらからも積極的に質問をすること。

1）　ジュリアに続いて各質問を発音してみよう。（▶動画２）

2）　今度は日本語を聞いてすぐに英語に訳してみよう。（▶動画３）

3）　質問と答えを交えながら、二人と会話をしてみよう。

　　　ダイアログ１：名前は？（▶動画４）

　　　ダイアログ２：どこに住んでいるか？通学方法は？（▶動画５）

　　　ダイアログ３：好きな食べ物は？好きなピザトッピングは？（▶動画６）

　　　ダイアログ４：趣味は？（▶動画７）

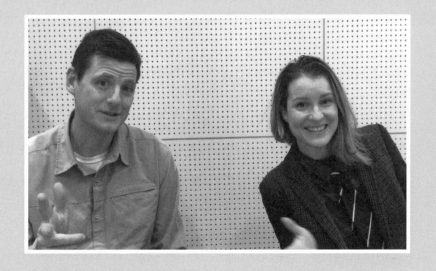

Lesson 6
X-ray / Diagnosis
レントゲン・診断

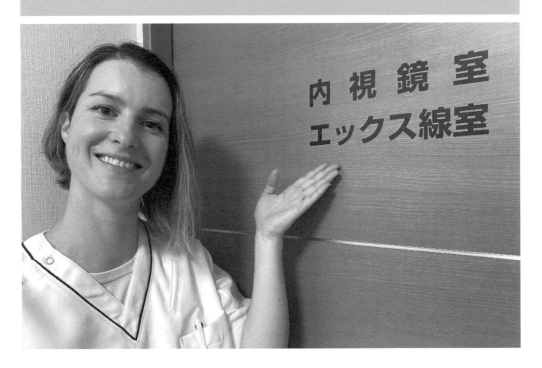

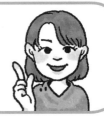
1 Core Terms
次の語を英語の場合は日本語に、日本語の場合は英語に直しなさい。

1. レントゲン   2. お腹   3. 金属の   4. 階

5. 判断する（j） 6. 詳細   7. object   8. receptionist

9. appendicitis 10. inflammation 11. appendix   12. operation

13. contact

2 Brian's Pronunciation Practice
動画の音声に続いてリピートしなさい。

3 Pronunciation Tips
動画の音声に続いて単語の発音練習をしなさい。

[xの発音] 1. x-ray　　2. appendix　　3. oxide　　4. examination　　5. xylitol

[注] oxide ＝酸化物　　xylitol ＝キシリトール

4 Core Phrases
次の英文を和訳しなさい。

1. We are going to take an x-ray of your stomach.

2. Make sure you do not have any metal objects on you.

3. Do you have any metal objects inside your body?

4. Be sure to give this file to the receptionist.

5. Judging from the tests, you have appendicitis.

6. We will get ready for an operation.

7. Is there anyone you can contact at home?

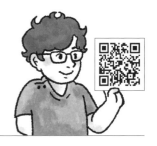

5 Quick Response
動画を見て日本語に対する英訳を瞬時に
口頭で言いなさい。瞬発力が大事です！

6 Warm-up

動画を見て、ブライアン先生が言う病院内の各エリアの名称を書きとりなさい。

1. 検査室   2. レントゲン室   3. 採血室

4. 男性用トイレ   5. 女性用トイレ   6. 多目的トイレ

7. 待合室   8. 売店   9. 会計

10. 受付

7 Workout with Julia

病院内の各場所への案内を動画で見て空欄を埋めなさい。
次に、字幕付きの動画を見てジュリアと一緒に発音しなさい。

1. (   )は(   )をまっすぐ進んで(   )に曲がってください。

2. (   )へは(   )で(   )階まで行ってください。

3. (   )は向かって(   )側の(   )番目の部屋です。

4. 最も近い (   ) は (   ) にあります。

5. (   ) はエレベーターホールの (   ) にあります。

6. ご家族とはこの (   ) の(   )でお会いになれます。

7. この (   ) の (   ) から電話をかけてください。

8. (   ) は (   ) 階にあります。

9. (   ) は1階の (   ) の横です。

8 Dialogs

動画を見て次の空欄を埋めなさい。

Dialog 1:（レントゲンを撮ります）

Nurse: Now we are going to take an x-ray of your stomach.

Patient: OK.

Nurse: Make sure you do not have any metal objects on you.

Patient: Alright. I'll (   )(   )(   ) (   ) and (   ).

Nurse:　Do you have any metal objects inside your body?

Patient:　What do you (　　　　　　　)(　　　　　　　)(　　　　　　　)
?

Nurse:　For example, clips, stents, pacemakers....

Patient:　Oh, I'm OK.

Nurse:　Be sure to give this file to the receptionist.

Patient:　So, how do I (　　　　　　)(　　　　　　)(　　　　　　)
(　　　　　　)(　　　　　　)?

Nurse:　Please take the elevator to the first floor.

Patient:　OK, thanks.

Dialog 2: (虫垂炎ですよ)

Doctor:　Mr. Bachman, judging from the test, you have appendicitis.

Patient:　(　　　　　　)(　　　　　　)(　　　　　　)?

Doctor:　It is inflammation of your appendix.

Patient:　Does it need to (　　　　　　)(　　　　　　)?

Doctor:　Yes, we will get ready for an operation this afternoon.

Patient:　Yipes!

(moments later)

Nurse:　Is there anyone you can contact at home?

Patient:　Yes, (　　　　　　)(　　　　　　)(　　　　　　)
(　　　　　　)(　　　　　　).

Nurse:　The doctor will explain the details to your wife.

Patient:　OK. I will (　　　　　　)(　　　　　　).

9 Listening Comprehension

「8」Dialogs の動画をもう一度見て巻末の Answer Sheet にある問題を
解きなさい。

10 Vocabulary Test

巻末の Answer Sheet の裏面にあるテストを受けなさい。

Lesson 7
Injection
注射

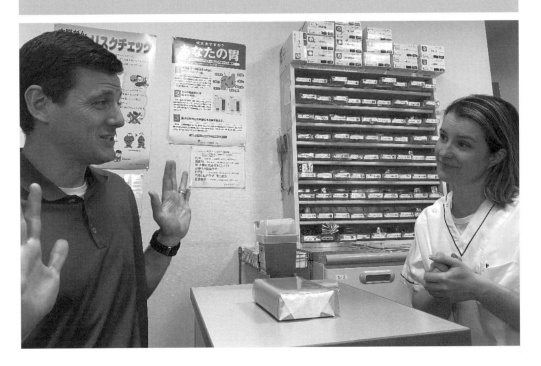

ナースカナのワンポイントアドバイス

In order to safely conduct this procedure, cooperation from the patient is necessary. Ask them to keep still and relax. In many cases, the injection is administered to relieve their symptoms. Explain how soon the medication will take effect. This will reassure the patients. For those new on the job, don't hesitate to ask senior nurses to accompany you during the procedure. At all times, stay calm.

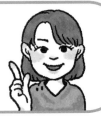

1 Core Terms
次の語を英語の場合は日本語に、日本語の場合は英語に直しなさい。

1. まだ（s）   2. 処方する   3. 注射（i）   4. 和らげる

5. アレルギー反応   6. 緩める（l）   7. a couple of ~   8. subside

9. immediately   10. alcohol wipes   11. right handed   12. get ready for ~

13. numbness   14. tingling

2 Brian's Pronunciation Practice
動画の音声に続いてリピートしなさい。

3 Pronunciation Tips
動画の音声に続いて単語の発音練習をしなさい。

［lとrの発音］ 1. light　　2. right　　3. lady　　4. ready　　5. lay　　6. ray

4 Core Phrases
次の英文を和訳しなさい。

1. I will give you an injection to relieve the pain.

2. Are you allergic to any medication?

3. Have you experienced any allergic reactions?

4. Are you right handed or left handed?

5. May I see your left arm?

6. Please relax and loosen your shoulders.

7. I will inject the medication.

5 Quick Response
動画を見て日本語に対する英訳を瞬時に
口頭で言いなさい。瞬発力が大事です！

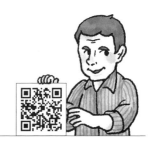

6 Warm-up
患者のアレルギーを尋ねる際にどのような質問をするべきか、
及びどのような回答が考えられるのかここで確認しなさい。

1. What are you allergic to?　あなたは何に対してアレルギーを持っていますか？
　 I am allergic to....（例）I am allergic to cats.　私は猫アレルギーです。

2. Do you have any allergies?　アレルギーはありますか？

I have....（例）I have peanut allergy.　私はナッツアレルギーです。

3. What are your symptoms?　あなたの症状は何ですか？

患者は痛みなど症状を抱えながら答えるので、文になっていないことが多々あります。重要なのは症状をしっかりと聞き取ることです。以下の症状を参考にしましょう。

itchiness　痒み	rashes　発疹	breathing trouble　呼吸困難
swollen eye lids　瞼の腫れ	red eyes　充血	itchy eyes　目の痒み
sneezing　くしゃみ	coughing　咳	nausea (vomiting)　吐き気（嘔吐）

 Workout with Julia
動画を見て問診票を日本語で記入しなさい。

	何に対してのアレルギー？	症状は？
1		
2		
3		
4		
5		
6		
7		
8		
9		
10		

 Dialogs
動画を見て次の空欄を埋めなさい。

Dialog 1:（痛み止めの注射を打ちます）

Nurse:　Mr. Bachman? Do you still have stomach pains?

Patient: Yes, (　　　　　　)(　　　　　　).

Nurse:　The doctor will prescribe an injection for the pain.

Patient: But, but...I (　　　　　　)(　　　　　　)(　　　　　　).

Nurse:　Don't worry, it will be over in a couple of seconds.

Patient: OK. How soon will it (   ) (   )
(   )?

Nurse: The pain should start to subside immediately.

Dialog 2: (どちらの腕にしますか？)

Nurse: I will give you an injection to relieve the pain.

Patient: Uh, OK.

Nurse: Are you allergic to any medication?

Patient: No, I am not.

Nurse: Have you experienced any allergic reactions to alcohol wipes?

Patient: No, I haven't.

Nurse: Are you right handed or left handed?

Patient: (   ) (   ) (   )
(   ).

Nurse: May I see your left arm?

It looks OK. I will get ready for the injection.

Please relax and loosen your shoulders.

Patient: OK.

Nurse: You will feel a slight pain.

Do you feel any numbness or tingling?

Patient: No.

Nurse: OK. I will inject the medication.

Nurse: We are finished.

I will remove the needle.

Press on this to stop the bleeding.

Patient: Thanks.

Listening Comprehension

「8」Dialogsの動画をもう一度見て巻末のAnswer Sheetにある問題を
解きなさい。

Patient Interview Practice

巻末のAnswer Sheetの裏面にある問題を解きなさい。

Lesson 8
Concerning the Operation
手術説明

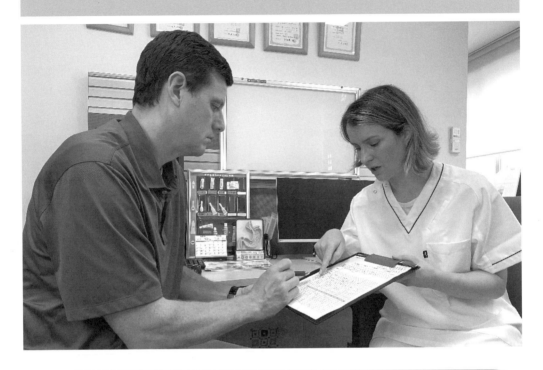

ナースカナのワンポイントアドバイス

Before an operation, the patient is concerned whether there will be any pain, how long will it take, or when they can get back to work. All of these uncertainties may cause a considerable amount of fear. In order to lighten this burden, it is our duty to respond to any kind of inquiry made by the patient.

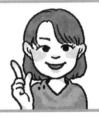

1 Core Terms
次の語を英語の場合は日本語に、日本語の場合は英語に直しなさい。

1. 手術
2. 説明する
3. 緊張した状態（n）

4. サインする
5. 質問
6. シャワーを浴びる（3語）

7. anesthesia
8. relieved
9. procedures
10. consent form

11. concerning
12. smoothly
13. rice porridge
14. wipe

2 Brian's Pronunciation Practice
動画の音声に続いてリピートしなさい。

3 Pronunciation Tips
動画の音声に続いて単語の発音練習をしなさい。

［bとvの発音］ 1. trouble　　2. nervous　　3. blood　　4. vein　　5. problem
6. relieved

4 Core Phrases
次の英文を和訳しなさい。

1. How do you feel?

2. You'll be under anesthesia.

3. You won't feel anything.

4. You need to sign a consent form.

5. Can you read Japanese?

6. Do you have any questions concerning the explanation?

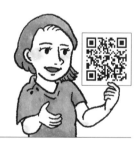

5 Quick Response
動画を見て日本語に対する英訳を瞬時に
口頭で言いなさい。瞬発力が大事です！

6 Warm-up
下の説明を読んで症状の期間や頻度の尋ね方の表現について理解しなさい。

症状がいつから始まったか、また症状の期間や頻度を患者に尋ねる際、以下のような
フレーズを使います。
1. いつから
　　When did the ~ start?　いつから~がありますか？

（例）When did the pain start? / When did the symptom start?

2. 期間

How long does ~ last?　どれくらいの間、~は続いていますか？

（例）How long does the itchiness last? / How long does the pain last?

3. 頻度（断続的か継続的か）

Is the ~ intermittent or constant?　~は断続的ですか、継続的ですか。

（例）Is the pain intermittent or constant? / The coughing is constant.（咳は継続的です。）

1～3の質問でよく使う症状も覚えておく必要があります。

pain　痛み	itchiness　痒み	dizziness　めまい
nausea　吐き気	coughing　咳	dullness　倦怠感

Workout with Julia

動画の問診を聞いて、患者の症状とそれがいつからで、
断続的なのか継続的なのかを以下の表に書きとりなさい。

	症状	いつから	断続的 or 継続 or その他
Case 1			
Case 2			
Case 3			
Case 4			
Case 5			
Case 6			

Dialogs

動画を見て次の空欄を埋めなさい。

Dialog 1:（同意書にサインをしてください）

Nurse:　Mr. Bachman. So, how do you feel?

Patient: I'm kind of (　　　　　　　　).

Nurse:　Don't worry.

Patient: I'm trying not to. Will it (　　　　　　　　　)?

Nurse:　You'll be under anesthesia, so you won't feel anything.

Patient: OK. I'm a bit (　　　　　　　) to hear that.

Nurse:　Before starting the procedures, you need to sign a consent form.

Patient: No problem.

Nurse:　So, here is the form. Can you read Japanese?

Patient: Uh, no....

Nurse:　OK. Here's what it says....

Dialog 2: (翌日はお粥しか食べられません)

Nurse:　Do you have any questions concerning the explanations?

Patient: Yes, I do. When can I (　　　　　　　)(　　　　　　　　) after the
operation?

Nurse:　If everything goes smoothly, you can eat lunch tomorrow.

Patient: (　　　　　　　)(　　　　　　　)(　　　　　　　) food can I
eat?

Nurse:　For tomorrow, you can only eat rice porridge.

Patient: When can I (　　　　　　)(　　　　　　　　)(　　　　　　　)?

Nurse:　Not tomorrow.

Patient: Oh....

Nurse:　I will wipe your body. You can start taking showers from the day after
tomorrow.

9 Listening Comprehension
「8」Dialogs の動画をもう一度見て巻末の Answer Sheet にある問題を
解きなさい。

10 Vocabulary Test
巻末の Answer Sheet の裏面にあるテストを受けなさい。

Lesson 9
After the Operation
術後

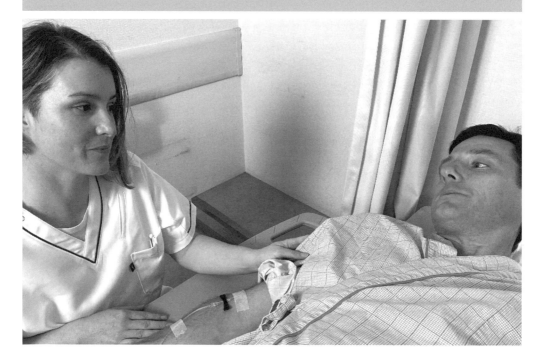

ナースカナのワンポイントアドバイス

Management of the patient's diet is also a part of our daily work. It is important to explain why there are diet restrictions before and after the operation. For example, the patient must cut down on sodium intake or even refrain from eating. In addition, informing how long the rehabilitation continues will encourage the patient and lead to better results.

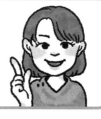

1 Core Terms
次の語を英語の場合は日本語に、日本語の場合は英語に直しなさい。

1. 血管	2. きつい (t)	3. リラックスする	4. ジュース
5. スープ	6. フルーツ	7. 加える	
8. intravenous infusion		9. insert	10. fluid
11. slight	12. tourniquet	13. digestion	14. broil

2 Brian's Pronunciation Practice
動画の音声に続いてリピートしなさい。

3 Pronunciation Tips
動画の音声に続いて単語の発音練習をしなさい。

［u:］ 1. juice　　2. fruit　　3. tube　　4. soup　　5. infusion

4 Core Phrases
次の英文を和訳しなさい。

1. I need to give you an intravenous infusion.

2. A small plastic tube is inserted into your vein.

3. It is necessary to give you fluids.

4. I am going to put a tourniquet on.

5. If it is too tight, let me know.

5 Quick Response
動画を見て日本語に対する英訳を瞬時に口頭で言いなさい。
瞬発力が大事です！

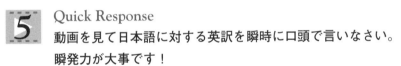

6 Warm-up
動画を見てブライアン先生に続いてリピートしなさい。次にもう一度動画を
見てブライアン先生の言った英単語を日本語で言いなさい。

stethoscope　聴診器	exam gloves　グローブ
blood pressure monitor　血圧計	electronic thermometer　電子体温計
cotton swab　綿棒［Q-tip ともいう］	dressing　包帯
saline　生理食塩水	tweezers　鑷子（せっし）
kidney tray　膿盆	syringe　注射器
sharps disposal　針捨て容器	tongue depressor　舌圧子

Workout with Julia

動画を見てナースジュリアの質問（What's this?／これは何ですか？）に
英語の文（This is ~ ／これは～です）で答えなさい。

写真の器具名を英語で書きなさい。

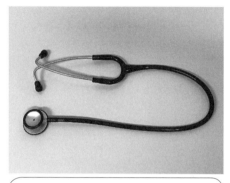

(1.)

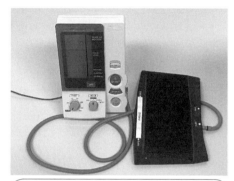

(2.)

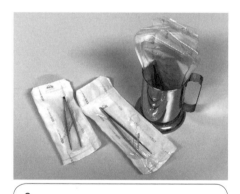

(3.)

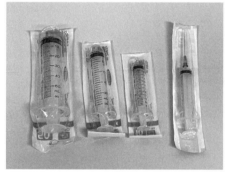

(4.)

 Dialogs

動画を見て次の空欄を埋めなさい。

Dialog 1: (点滴をします)

Nurse: I need to give you an intravenous infusion.

Patient: How are you going (　　　　　　)(　　　　　　)

(　　　　　　)?

Nurse: A small plastic tube is inserted into your vein.

Patient: I see.

Nurse:　It is necessary to give you fluids.

Patient: Will it be (　　　　　　　　)?

Nurse:　There is only a slight pain at the beginning.

Nurse:　I am going to put the tourniquet on now.

Nurse:　If it is too tight, let me know.

Patient: I am OK.

（all set）

Nurse:　Is everything OK?

Patient: I feel (　　　　　　　).

Dialog 2: (まずは消化に良い食事から)

Patient: So, what (　　　　　　　)(　　　　　　　)(　　　　　　　)

　　　　　eating here?

Nurse:　You will be eating foods that help digestion.

Patient: What kind of food (　　　　　　　)(　　　　　　)

　　　　　(　　　　　　　)?

Nurse:　You will start off with rice porridge, soup, and juice.

Patient: I see.

Nurse:　From day 3, rice, broiled fish, potato salad, and canned fruit will be added to

　　　　　the menu.

Patient: Oh boy, I can't wait!

Listening Comprehension
「8」Dialogsの動画をもう一度見て巻末のAnswer Sheetにある問題を
解きなさい。

Patient Interview Practice
巻末のAnswer Sheetの裏面にある問題を解きなさい。

Lesson 10
Dry Bath
清拭

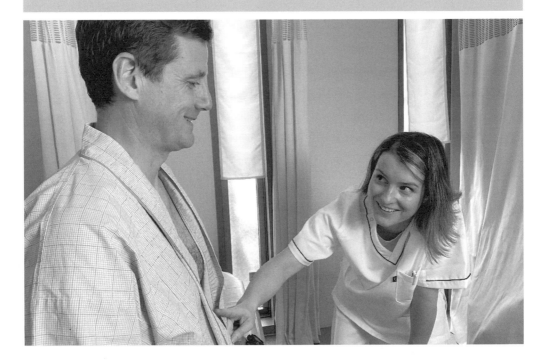

ナースカナのワンポイントアドバイス

A dry bath or bed bath is not only for keeping the patient's body clean. It is a chance to obtain information concerning the patient. By touching the body, you can tell if the patient has fever, rashes, swelling, dry skin, or even bed sores. This vital information is passed on to the physician as well as used to provide necessary nursing. However, keep in mind that this procedure can be embarrassing for the patient.

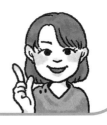

1 Core Terms
次の語を英語の場合は日本語に、日本語の場合は英語に直しなさい。

1. タオル	2. 予定する（s）	3. リハビリテーション	
4. シャツ	5. 縫い目	6. 痒い	7. correct
8. take off	9. rash	10. tummy	11. surgical tape

2 Brian's Pronunciation Practice
動画の音声に続いてリピートしなさい。

3 Pronunciation Tips
動画の音声に続いて単語の発音練習をしなさい。

[tʃ] 1. stitch   2. itch   3. catch   4. kitchen   5. pitcher

4 Core Phrases
次の英文を和訳しなさい。

1. Like I explained before, I can give you a dry bath.

2. I will wipe your body with a hot towel.

3. Let's do it after your rehabilitation.

4. Is it too hot?

5. Can you take your shirt off?

6. I'll have the doctor check it.

5 Quick Response
動画を見て日本語に対する英訳を瞬時に口頭で言いなさい。
瞬発力が大事です！

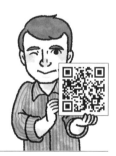

6 Warm-up
下の説明を読んで痛みの場所の尋ね方の表現について理解しなさい。

まずは患者さんにどこが痛むのかを訊く必要があります。
Where does it hurt? / Where is the pain?

上にあるhurtは「痛む」という動詞です。一方、painは「痛み」という名詞です。
両方とも一般的な英語の表現なので、患者さんに痛みの場所等を訊く際はこの英単語

を使うと良いでしょう。

ただし、患者さんからの答えでは痛みの種類によって他の表現が使われる可能性があります。なぜなら、英語には痛みの種類別にいくつかの呼び方が存在するからです。

pain　主に急性の激しい痛みを表す。
ache　主に鈍い持続的な痛みを表す。
sore　傷や炎症によるヒリヒリした痛みを表す。

これに伴い、痛みの答え方もいくつかのバリエーションが存在します。
体の部位ごとにそれぞれ練習してみましょう。

I have a 〜ache. / I have a pain in my 〜. / My 〜 hurts.

背中 back：I have a backache. / I have a pain in my back. / My back hurts.
お腹 stomach: I have a stomachache. / I have a pain in my stomach. / My stomach hurts.
頭 head: I have a headache. / I have a pain in my head. / My head hurts.
胸 chest: I have a chest ache. / I have a pain in my chest. / My chest hurts.
喉 throat: I have a sore throat. / I have a pain in my throat. / My throat hurts.

 Workout with Julia
**動画を見て患者の訴える痛みの場所と種類を日本語で
書きとりなさい。**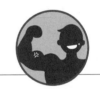

	痛みの場所	痛みの種類
Case 1		
Case 2		
Case 3		
Case 4		
Case 5		
Case 6		
Case 7		
Case 8		

8 Dialogs
動画を見て次の空欄を埋めなさい。

Dialog 1：（熱いタオルで体を拭きます）

Patient: So I can't (   ) (   ) (   ) today, right?

Nurse: That's correct. You just had an operation.
Like I explained before, I can give you a dry bath.

Patient: What was that?

Nurse: I will wipe your body with a hot towel.

Patient: Oh yes, right! Good idea...but I am (   )
(   ) (   ).

Nurse: No problem. Let's do it after your rehabilitation.

Dialog 2：（お腹に湿疹が）

Nurse: I will wipe your body.

Patient: Great.

Nurse: May I have your arm? Is it too hot?

Patient: No, it's (   ) (   ).

Nurse: Can you take your gown off?

Patient: I'll try...Oooh! (   ) (   )
(   ).

Nurse: OK. I'll help you.

(moments later)

Nurse: Hmmmm. You have rashes on your tummy. Does it itch?

Patient: No, it doesn't.

Nurse: It probably got red from the surgical tape. I'll have the doctor check it.

Patient: Thanks.

(moments later)

Patient: Wow. I feel (   ).

9 Listening Comprehension
「8」Dialogs の動画をもう一度見て巻末の Answer Sheet にある問題を
解きなさい。

---

10 Vocabulary Test
巻末の Answer Sheet の裏面にあるテストを受けなさい。

英会話コーナー 2

 身体や健康について英会話をしてみよう。

コツ❶ 質問に対して単語のみではなく、主語・動詞をつけて<u>文で答えるように心がける</u>。

例　質問　Do you have time now?
　　　　　今お時間ありますか？

　　回答　Yes.　✕
　　　　　はい。
　　　　　Yes, I do.　○
　　　　　はい、あります。

次の各質問に対する返事を完成させよう。（質問の太字が回答の主語・動詞に使われる）

●質問

Are you healthy?
あなたは健康ですか？

How many hours do you sleep?
あなたの睡眠時間は？

How tall are you?
あなたの身長は？

What is your blood pressure?
あなたの血圧は何ですか？

Are you experiencing any stress now?
ストレスを感じていますか？

Have you ever been on a diet?
ダイエットをしたことはありますか？

●回答

Yes, I am healthy. / No, I am not healthy.

I sleep ＿＿＿＿＿＿＿＿＿＿＿＿＿＿ hours.

I am ＿＿＿＿＿＿＿＿＿ centimeters tall.

My blood pressure is ＿＿＿＿ over ＿＿＿＿.

Yes, I am. / No, I'm not.

Yes, I have. / No, I have not.

コツ❷　こちらからも積極的に質問をすること。

1)　ジュリアに続いて各質問を発音してみよう。（▶動画２）

2)　今度は日本語を聞いてすぐに英語に訳してみよう。（▶動画３）

3)　質問と答えを交えながら、二人と会話をしてみよう。
　　ダイアログ１：あなたは健康ですか？（▶動画４）

　　　　　　あなたの睡眠時間は？

　　ダイアログ２：あなたの身長は？（▶動画５）

　　ダイアログ３：あなたの血圧は何ですか？（▶動画６）

　　　　　　ストレスを感じていますか？

　　　　　　ダイエットをしたことはありますか？

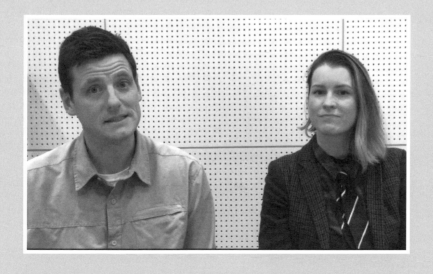

Lesson 11

Prescription

服薬指導

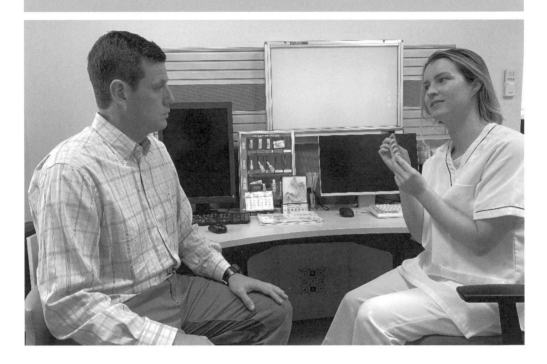

ナースカナのワンポイントアドバイス

Medication is necessary to regain the health of the patient. However, mistakes such as administering double the amount of medicine or forgetting to give a pill at the appointed time can hinder the effect of the treatment. In some cases, it can lead to serious consequences. We need to pay our utmost attention to information concerning the type, amount, and timing of the medication.

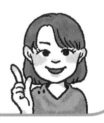

1 Core Terms
次の語を英語の場合は日本語に、日本語の場合は英語に直しなさい。

1. 服薬	2. 痛み止め	3. 錠剤（t）	4. 毎～（e）
5. 食事	6. 荒らす（u）	7. stomach	8. antibiotics
9. pill	10. course	11. leftovers	

2 Brian's Pronunciation Practice
動画の音声に続いてリピートしなさい。

3 Pronunciation Tips
動画の音声に続いて単語の発音練習をしなさい。

［ch の発音］1. each   2. scratch   3. stomach   4. ache   5. machine

4 Core Phrases
次の英文を和訳しなさい。

1. I will explain your medication.

2. Take 1 tablet, 3 times a day, after each meal.

3. They ［お薬］ will upset your stomach.

4. Be sure to take them after meals.

5. You will take these antibiotics for 1 week.

6. Be sure to finish the course.

7. Take it with water, not with coffee or juice.

5 Quick Response
動画を見て日本語に対する英訳を瞬時に口頭で言いなさい。
瞬発力が大事です！

6 Warm-up

患者への服薬指導の際に伝えるべき重要な情報は、「何を（What）」処方する
のか、「なぜ（Why）」服薬するのか、「いつ（When）」服薬するのか、
の3つです。各単語を「…」にあてはめて発音しなさい。

1. What

This medicine is....　このお薬は…です／This is....　これは…です

steroid　ステロイド　　　　　　　fever reducer　解熱剤　　painkiller　痛み止め

sleeping pills　睡眠導入剤　　　　anti-flatulent　整腸剤

allergy eye drops　アレルギー目薬

2. Why

It is to....　これは…のためです（toの後に続く動詞です）

treat　治療する　　reduce　減らす　　help　助ける　　relieve　和らげる

3. When

Apply... several times a day.　1日数回…を塗ってください

Take... pills (tablets) three times a day.　1日3回…錠を服用してください

twice a day　1日2回　　　before meals　食前　　　after each meal　毎食後

～するときはいつでも　whenever you have ～　　　就寝前に　before going to bed

7 Workout with Julia

動画を見て、服薬指導の際の「何を」、「なぜ」、「いつ」の
3つを聴き取って以下の表を英語もしくは日本語で埋めなさい。

	What	Why	When
(1)			
(2)			
(3)			
(4)			
(5)			
(6)			
(7)			

8 Dialogs
動画を見て次の空欄を埋めなさい。

Dialog 1：(痛み止めです…)

Nurse:　Mr. Bachman, I will explain your medication.
Patient: OK.
Nurse:　These are painkillers.
Patient: Right.
Nurse:　Take 1 tablet, 3 times a day, after each meal.
Patient: Can I take them (　　　　　　)(　　　　　　)?
Nurse:　They will upset your stomach.
　　　　Be sure to take them after meals.
Patient: I'll (　　　　　　)(　　　　　　).
Nurse:　This is stomach medicine.
Patient: I see.
Nurse:　Take 1 tablet, 3 times a day, after each meal…same as pain killers.
Patient: OK.

Dialog 2：(必ず飲み切ってくださいね…)

Nurse:　Mr. Bachman, here are your antibiotics.
　　　　Be sure to take 1 pill after breakfast only.
Patient: (　　　　　　)(　　　　　　) in the morning?
Nurse:　That's right. You will take these antibiotics for 1 week.
Patient: 1 week?
Nurse:　Yes. Be sure to finish the course.
Patient: No (　　　　　　)?
Nurse:　No leftovers.
　　　　Also, take it with water, not with coffee or juice.
Patient: No (　　　　　　)(　　　　　　)?
Nurse:　No soft drinks.

9 Listening Comprehension

「8」Dialogsの動画をもう一度見て巻末のAnswer Sheetにある問題を
解きなさい。

10 Patient Interview Practice

巻末のAnswer Sheetの裏面にある問題を解きなさい。

Lesson 12
Common Cold
風邪

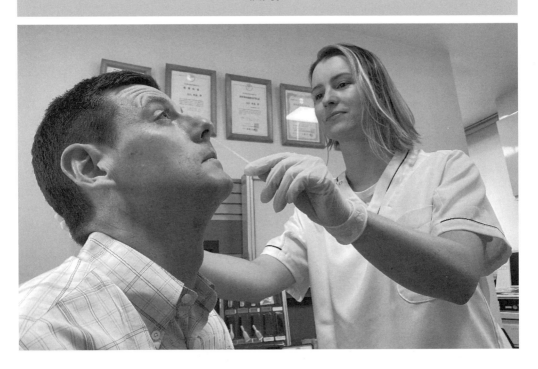

The common cold is prevalent year round. However, as the cold weather approaches, cases suddenly increase. Everyone has experienced the symptoms of colds such as sore throat, stuffy nose, runny nose, coughs, mild headaches, sneezing, fever, and mild body aches. The best remedy for the common cold is to keep warm and get plenty of rest...and of course, do not forget to stay hydrated.

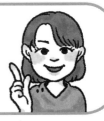

1 Core Terms
次の語を英語の場合は日本語に、日本語の場合は英語に直しなさい。

1. 風邪　　　2. 症状　　　3. 熱 (f)　　　4. 咳

5. インフルエンザ (f)　　　6. インフルエンザ (i)　　　7. 結果

8. run　　　9. constantly　　　10. appetite　　　11. bite（名詞）

12. nostril　　　13. uncomfortable　　　14. support　　　15. tissue paper

2 Brian's Pronunciation Practice
動画の音声に続いてリピートしなさい。

3 Pronunciation Tips
動画の音声に続いて単語の発音練習をしなさい。

［pの発音］ 1. symptom   2. appetite   3. support   4. paper   5. put

4 Core Phrases
次の英文を和訳しなさい。

1. When did the cough start?

2. How is your appetite?

3. We will do an influenza test.

4. I will put this Q-Tip in your nostril.［Q-Tipはcotton swabともいう］

5. It might feel uncomfortable for a few seconds.

6. I will support the back of your head with my hand.

7. Please wait 30 minutes for the result.

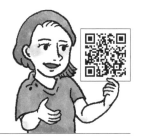

5 Quick Response
動画を見て日本語に対する英訳を瞬時に
口頭で言いなさい。瞬発力が大事です！

6 Warm-up
次の英語を和訳しなさい。

1. capsule

2. tablet

3. powdered medicine

4. syrup

5. ointment

6. eye drop

7. lozenge

8. suppository

9. compress

7 Workout with Julia
Part 1
動画を見てナースジュリアの質問（What's this? / これは何ですか？）
に英語の文（This is ~ / これは～です）で答えなさい。

Part 2
次に別の動画を見て以下の英文の空欄を埋めなさい。

1. このカプセルを1回2錠、1日3回、食後に服用してください。

   Take 2 (   ), three times a day, after each meal.
2. このタブレットを1回1錠お休みになる前に飲んでください。

   Take 1 (   ), once a day, before bedtime.
3. この粉薬を1回1包、食間に飲んでください。

   Take this (   )(   ) between meals.
4. この水薬を1回スプーン1杯分毎食後に飲んでください。

   Take one spoonful of this (   ) after each meal.
5. この塗り薬を1日に数回塗ってください。

   Apply this (   ) several times a day.
6. かゆい時にこの目薬を差してください。

   Use this (   )(   ) when it is itchy.

8 Dialogs
動画を見て次の空欄を埋めなさい。

Dialog 1：（風邪かも…）
Nurse:　What seems to be the problem?

Patient: I seem to have (   )(   )

　　　　　(   ).

Nurse: What are the symptoms?

Patient: I think I am (   )(   )(   ).

Nurse: Are there any other symptoms?

Patient: I am (   )(   ).

Nurse: When did the cough start?

Patient: It started last night.

Nurse: ...and how is your appetite?

Patient: I don't feel like eating. I haven't (   )(   )
(   ) since yesterday.

Nurse: I see.

Dialog 2：（少しがまんして下さいね…）

Nurse: You might have the flu.

Patient: Oh my gosh!

Nurse: We will do an influenza test.

Patient: (   )(   )(   ) test will that
be?

Nurse: I will put this Q-Tip in your nostril.

Patient: Will it hurt?

Nurse: It might feel uncomfortable for a few seconds.

(moments later)

Nurse: I will support the back of your head with my hand...hold on.
Here you are. (handing tissue paper)

Patient: Thanks.

Nurse: We are finished.
Please wait 30 minutes for the results.

9 Listening Comprehension
「8」Dialogs の動画をもう一度見て巻末の Answer Sheet にある問題を
解きなさい。

10 Vocabulary Test
巻末の Answer Sheet の裏面にあるテストを受けなさい。

Lesson 13
Influenza
インフルエンザ

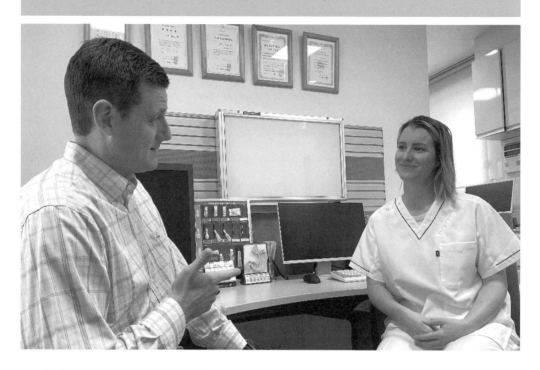

ナースカナのワンポイントアドバイス

With the approach of the winter season, there is a steady increase of influenza cases. It is important for nurses to protect themselves from catching the flu. In addition, we must not become a carrier of the virus and spread it to our patients. Be sure to wash your hands, gargle, and conduct disinfection of surfaces. We are fighting an invisible enemy. This is why the utmost care is necessary.

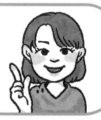

1 Core Terms
次の語を英語の場合は日本語に、日本語の場合は英語に直しなさい。

1. 陽性　　　　2. 撒き散らす　　3. 体温

4. 距離を置く（2語）　5. （マスクを）着ける

6. 栄養　　　7. sick leave　　8. prescribe　　9. fluid

10. rest　　　11. recommend　　12. digestion　　13. afterwards

2 Brian's Pronunciation Practice
動画の音声に続いてリピートしなさい。

3 Pronunciation Tips
動画の音声に続いて単語の発音練習をしなさい。

[tion の発音] 　1. nutri<u>tion</u>　　2. diges<u>tion</u>　　3. medica<u>tion</u>　　4. prescrip<u>tion</u>
　　　　　　　5. opera<u>tion</u>

4 Core Phrases
次の英文を和訳しなさい。

1. You may not go to work.

2. Try to stay away from others as much as possible.

3. Be sure to wear a mask at all times.

4. Be sure to take fluids such as sports drinks.

5. Be sure to rest well and get nutrition.

6. Take food that helps your digestion.

7. Be sure to keep warm.

8. Get a lot of sleep.

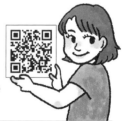

5 Quick Response
動画を見て日本語に対する英訳を瞬時に口頭で言いなさい。
瞬発力が大事です！

6 Warm-up
下の説明を読んで、痛みの程度の表現について理解しなさい。

痛みの程度

痛みの場所が分かったら、次はその程度を訊いてみましょう。

痛みの程度の表現として以下の3つは最低限覚えておきましょう。

- 激しい痛み　severe pain
- 軽い痛み　mild pain
- 我慢できる程度の痛み　tolerable pain

痛みの程度は英語で "the extent of the pain" ですが、痛みの程度を訊く際はその度合いを数値化して答えてもらう質問文が有効です。

10 being most severe, on a scale of 0 to 10 how would you rate your pain?
「10を最も激しい痛みとして、0から10で痛みを表すとどうなりますか？」
もう少し簡易的にすると、
Please rate your pain on a scale of one to ten.
「1から10で痛みを表してください。」

この数値化して答えてもらう方法は痛みの度合い以外も疲労の度合い、痒みの度合いなどで応用可能です。

7 Workout with Julia

Part 1の動画を見て、以下の表を英語もしくは日本語で埋めなさい。
Part 2の動画を見てナースジュリアに続いてリピートしなさい。

	Rate of pain（数値）	Nature of pain（性質）	Movement of pain（移動）
Case 1			
Case 2			
Case 3			

8 Dialogs

動画を見て次の空欄を埋めなさい。

Dialog 1: (陽性でした…)

Nurse:　What did the doctor say?

Patient: I (   ) (   ) for influenza.

Nurse: That is too bad.

Patient: What should I do? Can I go to work?

Nurse: You may not go to work. You don't want to spread your flu to others.

Patient: I see. Then, I will (   ) my boss (   )
           (   ) (   ).

           When can I go back to work?

Nurse: Usually, 48 hours after your temperature returns to normal.

Patient: OK. How about meeting other people?

Nurse: Try to stay away from others as much as possible.

           Also, be sure to wear a mask at all times.

Dialog 2: (消化によい食べ物を…)

Patient: What kind of (   ) will I (   )?

Nurse: We will prescribe medication.

Patient: I see.

Nurse: And please be sure to take fluids such as sports drinks.

Patient: OK.

Nurse: Also, be sure to rest well and get nutrition.

Patient: What kind of food is (   )?

Nurse: Take food that helps your digestion.

Patient: What about (   ) (   )?

Nurse: You may take showers but be sure to keep warm afterwards.

Patient: OK, I'll try.

Nurse: Finally, forget about your work and get a lot of sleep.

Patient: That's not bad!

9　Listening Comprehension

「8」Dialogs の動画をもう一度見て巻末の Answer Sheet にある問題を
解きなさい。

10　Patient Interview Practice

巻末の Answer Sheet の裏面にある問題を解きなさい。

Lesson 14
External Injury
外傷

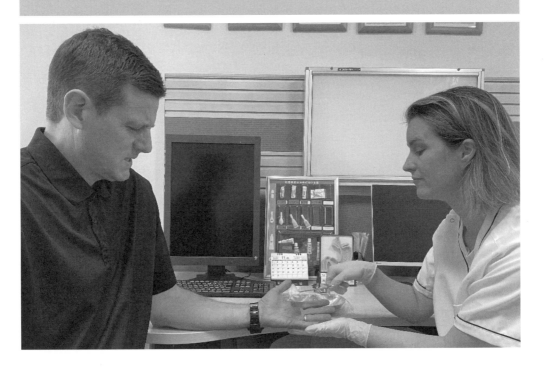

ナースカナのワンポイントアドバイス

External injuries occur when a person is involved in an accident or falls down. The injury could be minor such as a scrape. However, in some cases, it could be life threatening. The pain and bleeding may cause the patient to panic. In some cases, the sight of blood can make the patient faint. No matter what the reaction is, be sure to stay calm and conduct the necessary procedures.

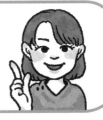

1 Core Terms
次の語を英語の場合は日本語に、日本語の場合は英語に直しなさい。

1. 転ぶ	2. 膝	3. すりむく	4. 出血する
5. 消毒する	6. ガーゼ	7. slip	8. pavement
9. bruise	10. bone	11. site	12. sting
13. remove			

2 Brian's Pronunciation Practice
動画の音声に続いてリピートしなさい。

3 Pronunciation Tips
動画の音声に続いて単語の発音練習をしなさい。

[ɔ] 1. g<u>au</u>ze   2. f<u>a</u>ll   3. l<u>o</u>ng   4. th<u>ou</u>ght   5. t<u>a</u>lk

4 Core Phrases
次の英文を和訳しなさい。

1. How did it happen?

2. Let's take a look at your knee.

3. I will clean the bruise.

4. I will have the doctor check it.

5. I will disinfect the site.

6. It may sting a little.

7. Do not remove the gauze.

5 Quick Response
動画を見て日本語に対する英訳を瞬時に
口頭で言いなさい。瞬発力が大事です！

6 Warm-up

患者さんは様々な種類の痛みを訴えかけてきます。その呼び方を知っておくことが大切です。体の各部の名称を日本語に訳しなさい。

1. neck
2. temple
3. shoulder
4. chest

5. stomach
6. upper arm
7. elbow
8. forearm

9. wrist
10. palm
11. thigh
12. knee

13. shin
14. calf
15. ankle
16. back

17. spine

7 Workout with Julia

動画を見てナースジュリアの質問（What's this? / これは何ですか？）に英語の文（This is the〜 / これは〜です）で答えなさい。

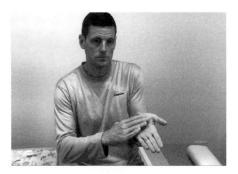
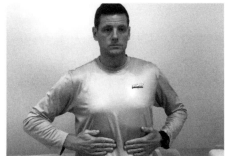
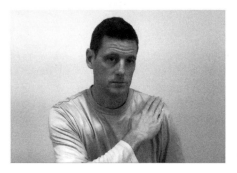
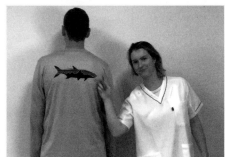

8 Dialogs
動画を見て次の空欄を埋めなさい。

Dialog 1：（自転車がすべって…）

Nurse:　What seems to be the problem?

Patient: I (　　　　　　　　) and (　　　　　　　　) my (　　　　　　　　).

Nurse:　How did it happen?

Patient: My bicycle slipped and I (　　　　　　　　) my knee (　　　　　　)
　　　　the pavement.

Nurse:　Did you hit your head or any other part of your body?

Patient: I didn't hit my head...but I (　　　　　　　) my hand.

Nurse:　I see. First, let's take a look at your knee.

Patient: Awww! It's (　　　　　　　)!

Nurse:　Don't worry, I will clean the bruise and have the doctor check it.

Dialog 2：（傷を消毒しますね…）

Nurse:　The x-ray shows there were no broken bones.

Patient: Oh, that is a (　　　　　　　)!

Nurse:　So, I will disinfect the site.

Patient: Will it hurt?

Nurse:　It may sting a little but you will be OK.

(moments later)

Patient: Can I take a shower today?

Nurse:　No. Please wait until tomorrow.

Patient: Do I (　　　　　　　) tomorrow?

Nurse:　Yes. I will check your bruise again.
　　　　Until then, do not remove the gauze.

9 Listening Comprehension
「8」Dialogs の動画をもう一度見て巻末の Answer Sheet にある問題を
解きなさい。

10 Vocabulary Test
巻末の Answer Sheet の裏面にあるテストを受けなさい。

Lesson 15
Loss of Appetite
食欲不振

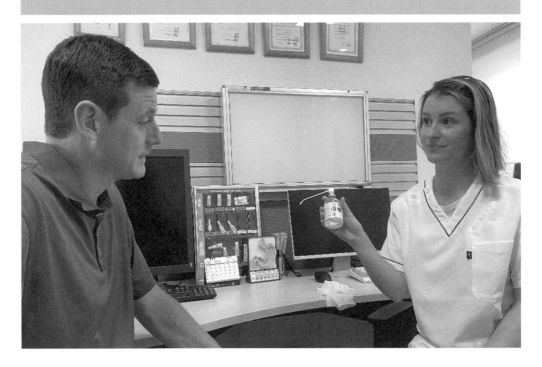

ナースカナのワンポイントアドバイス

Eating plays a key role in our overall health and well-being. That is why loss of appetite can become a serious problem. It is our role to try and find the cause and to consult with the physician or nutritionist. Think about what kind of food would be most appropriate for the patient. The texture, hot or cold foods, portion sizes, and choice of utensils are some of the things that we can consider.

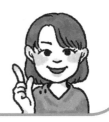

1 Core Terms
次の語を英語の場合は日本語に、日本語の場合は英語に直しなさい。

---

1. 食欲　　　　　2. 吐き気　　　　3. ストレス　　　4. 大変な（t）

5. プレッシャー　6. 検査する　　　7. heartburn　　8. blood sample

9. urine sample　10. endoscope　　11. anesthetic spray

Brian's Pronunciation Practice
動画の音声に続いてリピートしなさい。

Pronunciation Tips
動画の音声に続いて単語の発音練習をしなさい。

［ssの発音］1. stress　　2. pressure　　3. loss　　4. itchiness　　5. dessert

4 Core Phrases
次の英文を和訳しなさい。

1. Since when?

2. Do you have any nausea?

3. Is there anything that you can eat?

4. Are you experiencing any stress now?

5. We will do some tests.

6. We will take a blood sample and a urine sample.

7. We will also take an X-ray and a CT scan.

8. We will examine with an endoscope.

 Quick Response
動画を見て日本語に対する英訳を瞬時に
口頭で言いなさい。瞬発力が大事です！

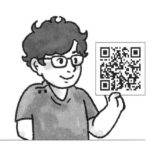

6 Warm-up
患者への服薬指導の際に伝えるべき重要な情報は、「何を（What）」処方する
のか、「なぜ（Why）」服薬するのか、「いつ（When）」服薬するのか、
の3つです。Lesson 11の復習もかねて練習しなさい。

1. What

This medicine is....　このお薬は…です／This is....　これは…です

以下の薬を「…」に当てはめて練習しなさい。

acid reducing drug　胃酸抑制剤　　　　　anti-allergic medicine　抗アレルギー薬

nitrate　舌下剤　※nitro vasodilator sublingual formulation（ニトロ系血管拡張薬）

an inhaler　吸入器　※asthma puffer 喘息吸入薬

burn cream　やけど軟膏（ワセリン）　　compress　湿布　　laxative　下剤

2. Why

It is to....　これは…のためです。

toの後に続く動詞です。

make it easy to ～　～しやすくする　　　decrease　減らす

It is for(症状).　これは(症状)のためです。

3. When

Inhale...three times a day.　1日3回…を吸入してください。

～の時　when ～　　シャワーの後　after showering　　就寝前に　before sleeping

 Workout with Julia
動画を見て、服薬指導の際の「何を」、「なぜ」、「いつ」の
3つを聴き取って以下の表を埋めなさい。

	What	Why	When
(1)			
(2)			
(3)			
(4)			
(5)			
(6)			
(7)			

Dialogs
動画を見て次の空欄を埋めなさい。

Dialog 1: (ストレスを感じていますか？)

Nurse: What seems to be the problem?

Patient: I seem to have (   ) my (   ).

Nurse: Since when?

Patient: For about (   )(   )(   )
(   ).

Nurse: Do you have any nausea?

Patient: I do not have any nausea but I have (   ).

Nurse: Is there anything you can eat?

Patient: I can eat (   ).

Nurse: Are you experiencing any stress now?

Patient: I am having a (   )(   ) at work. I feel a lot
of (   ).

Dialog 2: (色々な検査)

Nurse: Mr. Bachman, we will do some tests.

Patient: (   )(   )(   ) tests will you
do?

Nurse: Today, we will take a blood sample and urine sample.

Patient: I see.

Nurse: We will also take an x-ray and a CT scan.

Patient: Will that be all?

Nurse: There is one more. Next week, we will examine you with an endoscope.

Patient: What is that?

Nurse: It is a camera to look inside your stomach.

Patient: Ugh. (   )(   ).

Nurse: It is, but we will use some anesthetic spray.

 ## Listening Comprehension
「8」Dialogsの動画をもう一度見て巻末のAnswer Sheetにある問題を
解きなさい。

 ## Patient Interview Practice
巻末のAnswer Sheetの裏面にある問題を解きなさい。

Listening Comprehension

Dialog 1
Q1. What is the patient's problem?

Q2. How will he get to the clinic?

Dialog 2
Q1. Is the patient insured?

Q2. What did the nurse ask him to do?

Dialog 3
Q1. When will he be called?

Warm-up

括弧に英単語を補って、下の地図の矢印の通りに道案内をしなさい。

① (   )(   ) of the (   ) exit of the station.
   (   )(   ) and (   )(   )
   the hamburger shop. (   )(   ) at the barber shop.
   (   )(   ) and you will find the clinic (   )
   (   )(   )(   ).

② Go straight (   ) the river. Turn east (   ) the tall tree.
   (   )(   ) the shrine and turn right (   )
   the restaurant. (   )(   ) the police station and turn left
   (   ) the hotel. The clinic is (   )(   )
   (   ).

③ Kinpodo is located (   )(   ) this clinic. Go out of
   the clinic and turn right. Next, turn right (   )(   )
   (   ) of the hotel. Go straight and go past the police station. Turn right
   (   )(   )(   ) and (   )
   (   )(   ) a school. Turn left and go straight.
   (   )(   )(   ) Kinpodo on your left.

Listening Comprehension

Dialog 1

Q1. What kind of illness did the patient have last year?

Q2. What kind of surgery did he have a few years ago?

Dialog 2

Q1. Where is the pain?

Q2. What are the symptoms besides pain?

Vocabulary Test

次の語を英語にしなさい。

1. もう一度

2. 病気（ i ）

3. 病院

4. 前に（b）

5. ここ最近（c）

6. アレルギー

7. 深刻な（s）

8. 手術（o）

9. 投薬

10. 症状

Listening Comprehension

Dialog 1

Q1. What is the patient's temperature?

Q2. What is the patient's normal temperature?

Dialog 2

Q1. What is the patient's pulse rate?

Q2. What is the normal pulse rate for adults?

Patient Interview (1)

動画を見て、下の表を完成させなさい。

	箇所	症状
1		
2		
3		
4		
5		

Listening Comprehension

Dialog 1

Q1. What did the nurse wrap around the patient's arm?

Q2. What was his blood pressure?

Dialog 2

Q1. What was the patient's blood pressure?

Q2. Why was the blood pressure so high?

Vocabulary Test

次の語を英語にしなさい。

1. 測る（t）

2. テーブル

3. 秒

4. 圧迫する（s）

5. 外す（r）

6. （組んだ足などを）戻す

7. 血圧

8. カフ（腕巻き）

9. 圧迫する

10. 好む（p）

Listening Comprehension

Dialog 1

Q1. How should the patient make his fist?

Q2. What did the nurse do before inserting the needle?

Dialog 2

Q1. What must the patient do first when collecting the urine?

Q2. How much urine is necessary?

［注］鋭い＝sharp
　　 鈍い＝dull
　　 焼けるような＝burning
　　 ずきずきする＝throbbing（ドクドクと拍動するような痛み）
　　 ガンガンする＝pounding（打たれているような痛み：ひどい頭痛など）
　　 キューッとする＝squeezing（絞られるような、締め付けられるような痛み：胸部痛など）
　　 締め付けるような、差し込むような＝cramping（生理痛やこむら返りなど）
　　 刺すような＝stabbing
　　 ビーンと電気が走るような＝shooting
　　 割れるような＝splitting
　　 ぴりぴりうずくような＝tingling
　　 ちくっとする＝pricking
　　 しくしくする、しつこく感じる＝nagging

Patient Interview (2)

動画を見て、下の表を完成させなさい。

	箇所	症状
1		
2		
3		
4		
5		

Listening Comprehension

Dialog 1

Q1. What metal objects did the patient have on him?

Q2. How do you get to the x-ray room?

Dialog 2

Q1. What is the diagnosis?

Q2. When will the operation take place?

Vocabulary Test

次の語を英語にしなさい。

1. レントゲン

2. お腹

3. 金属の

4. 判断する（j）

5. 詳細

6. 受付

7. 虫垂炎

8. 炎症

9. 盲腸

10. 手術

Listening Comprehension

Dialog 1

Q1. What will the doctor prescribe for the pain?

Q2. How soon will the pain subside?

Dialog 2

Q1. Does the patient have any allergies?

Q2. Which arm did the nurse inject the medication?

Patient Interview (3)

動画を見て、下の表を完成させなさい。

	箇所	症状
1		
2		
3		
4		
5		

Listening Comprehension

Dialog 1

Q1. What is the patient worried about?

Q2. What does the patient need to sign before the operation?

Dialog 2

Q1. When can the patient start eating?

Q2. What will the patient eat on the next day after the operation?

Vocabulary Test

次の語を英語にしなさい。

1.　手術

2.　説明する

3.　緊張した状態（n）

4.　サインする

5.　質問（q）

6.　麻酔

7.　同意書（2 語）

8.　〜に関して（c）

9.　円滑に

10.　拭く（w）

Listening Comprehension

Dialog 1

Q1. How did the nurse explain an intravenous infusion?

Q2. Why is the intravenous infusion necessary?

Dialog 2

Q1. What kind of food will the patient eat?

Q2. What kind of food will the patient eat from day 3?

Patient Interview (4)

動画を見て、下の表を完成させなさい。

	箇所	症状
1		
2		
3		
4		
5		

Listening Comprehension

Dialog 1

Q1. How will the nurse give a dry bath?

Q2. When will she give the patient the dry bath?

Dialog 2

Q1. What did the patient have on his stomach?

Q2. What probably caused it?

Vocabulary Test

次の語を英語にしなさい。

1. タオル

2. 予定する（s）

3. リハビリテーション

4. シャツ

5. 縫い目

6. 痒い

7. 正しい（c）

8. 湿疹

9. お腹（t）

10. 外科用テープ（2語）

Listening Comprehension

Dialog 1

Q1. What is the prescription for the painkillers?

Q2. What is the prescription for the stomach medicine?

Dialog 2

Q1. What is the prescription for the antibiotics?

Q2. What should the patient take the antibiotics with?

Patient Interview (5)

動画を見て、下の表を完成させなさい。

	箇所	症状
1		
2		
3		
4		
5		

Listening Comprehension

Dialog 1

Q1. What are the symptoms?

Q2. How is the patient's appetite?

Dialog 2

Q1. What kind of influenza test will the patient take?

Q2. How long should the patient wait for the result?

Vocabulary Test

次の語を英語にしなさい。

1. 風邪

2. 熱（f）

3. 咳

4. インフルエンザ（i）

5. 結果

6. 絶え間なく

7. 食欲

8. 鼻孔

9. 不快な

10. 支える

Listening Comprehension

Dialog 1

Q1. What was the result of the test?

Q2. When can the patient go back to work?

Dialog 2

Q1. What kind of drinks are recommended?

Q2. What kind of food is recommended?

Patient Interview (6)

動画を見て、下の表を完成させなさい。

	箇所	症状
1		
2		
3		
4		
5		

Listening Comprehension

Dialog 1

Q1. How did the patient hurt his knee?

Q2. What will the nurse do before the doctor checks?

Dialog 2

Q1. What is the result of the x-ray?

Q2. When can the patient take a shower?

Vocabulary Test

次の語を英語にしなさい。

1. 転ぶ

2. 膝

3. すりむく

4. 出血する

5. 消毒する

6. ガーゼ

7. 傷口（b）

8. 骨

9. 患部（s）

10. チクッとする（s）

Listening Comprehension

Dialog 1

Q1. When did the patient lose his appetite?

Q2. Why is the patient experiencing stress?

Dialog 2

Q1. What kind of samples will be collected?

Q2. What is an endoscope?

Patient Interview (7)

動画を見て、下の表を完成させなさい。

	箇所	症状
1		
2		
3		
4		
5		

QRコードで動画が見られる！ 看護英語ワークブック

2021年3月15日　第1版 第1刷 ©

著　者	藤田淳一　FUJITA, Junichi
	岡 隼人　OKA, Hayato
発行者	宇山閑文
発行所	株式会社金芳堂
	〒606-8425 京都市左京区鹿ケ谷西寺ノ前町34番地
	振替　01030-1-15605
	電話　075-751-1111（代）
	https://www.kinpodo-pub.co.jp/
組版・装丁	HON DESIGN
イラスト	角 一葉
印刷・製本	モリモト印刷株式会社

落丁・乱丁本は直接小社へお送りください．お取替え致します．

Printed in Japan
ISBN978-4-7653-1853-2